AF440109

Pharmaceutical Analysis:
A Practical Manual

Pharmaceutical Analysis:
A Practical Manual

Editors

Dr. Randhir Singh Dahiya

Navpreet Kaur

Lalit Kishore

M.M. College of Pharmacy,
Maharishi Markandeshwar University,
Mullana-Ambala, Haryana-133207

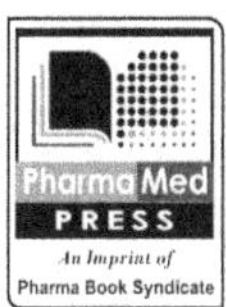

PharmaMed Press

An imprint of Pharma Book Syndicate

A unit of BSP Books Pvt. Ltd.

4-4-309/316, Giriraj Lane,

Sultan Bazar, Hyderabad - 500 095.

Pharmaceutical Analysis: A Practical Manual *by*

Dr. Randhir Singh Dahiya, Navpreet Kaur and Lalit Kishore

© 2016, *by Publisher*

Published by

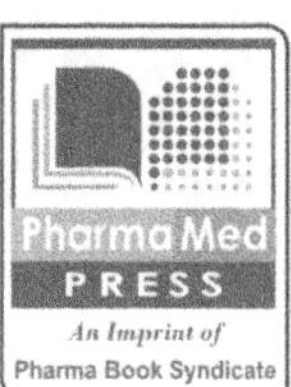

PharmaMed Press

An imprint of Pharma Book Syndicate

A unit of BSP Books Pvt. Ltd.

4-4-309/316, Giriraj Lane, Sultan Bazar, Hyderabad - 500 095.
Phone: 040-23445605, 23445688; Fax: 91+40-23445611
E-mail: info@pharmamedpress.com

ISBN: 978-93-5230-110-2 (HB)

PREFACE

Analytical chemistry has played a major role in the modernization of drug discovery and development. Traditionally viewed as a service industry, the analytical department has become the significant partner in the drug development. Testing a pharmaceutical product involves chemical, physical and sometimes microbiological analyses. It has been estimated that £10 billion is spent each year on analyses in the UK alone and such analytical processes can be found in industries as diverse as those producing food, beverages, cosmetics, detergents, metals, paints, water, agrochemicals, biotechnological products and pharmaceuticals. Presently, Pharmaceutical analysis involves a series of process for identification, determination, quantification and purification of a compound, separation of the components of a solution or mixture, or determination of structure of chemical compounds. Pharmaceutical companies rely upon both qualitative and quantitative chemical analysis to ensure that the raw material used to meet all the desired specifications and also to check the quality of the final product. Rapid advances have been made in many analytical techniques over the past few decades. The science and technology utilized today, coupled with the new regulations that are now binding, have made pharmaceutical analysis much more complicated compared to what it was as ten years before. The pharmaceutical analyst plays a major role in assuring identity, safety, efficacy, purity and quality of a drug product. With such large amounts of money being spent on analytical quality control, great importance must be placed on providing accurate and precise analyses. Thus it is appropriate to begin a book on the topic of pharmaceutical analysis by considering, at a basic level, the criteria which are used to judge the quality of an analysis. We believe that the valuable information presented in this manual will be found useful by those involved in various aspects of pharmaceutical analysis as they relate to production and control, new drug development, teaching or regulation.

- Authors

ACKNOWLEDGEMENT

It is a great privilege to express our sagacious sense of gratitude and admiration toward our esteemed venerable to Sh. Tarsem Kumar Garg, Chancellor, Maharishi Markandeshwar University, Mullana, Ambala. He has been a moving spirit behind this uphill task.

This book would not have been successful without noted help from our colleagues and Friends Dr. Anurag Kuhad, Dr. Jitender Bariwal, Dr. Mahender Bisnoi, Mr. Nikhil Tundwal, Mr. Sumit Wadhwa, Mr. Sameer, Mr. Harpeet Singh, Mr. Parvez Quarishi, Dr. Abhay Asthana, Dr. Gyati Shilakari, Mr. Shishant and Mr. Girish Gupta.

Personally, we are grateful to **our family** for their encouragement, support and the blessing.

We are thankful to **BS Publications**, for earliest possible publication of our book.

- Authors

CONTENTS

Chapter – 5

Non-aqueous Titration...92

Chapter – 6

Complexometric Titrations 119

Chapter – 9

Diazotization Titration 153

Experiment 9.1

Experiment 9.2

Chapter – 10

Conductometric Titrations..................................161

Experiment 10.1

Experiment 10.2

Chapter – 11

Flame Photometry..................................168

Experiment 11.1

Chapter – 12

Polarimetry 176

Experiment 12.1

Experiment 12.2

Chapter – 13

Chapter – 14

Chapter – 15

Chapter – 16

Chapter – 20

Infrared Spectrophotometry 264

Experiment 20.5

Chapter – 21

High Performance Liquid Chromatography 281

Experiment 21.1

Introduction

Analytical chemistry is the study of the separation, identification, and quantification of the chemical components of natural and synthetic materials. Qualitative analysis gives an indication of the identity of the chemical species in the sample and quantitative analysis determines the amount of one or more of these components.

Titrimetric Analysis

Titrimetric methods of analysis are capable of rapid and convenient analyte determinations with high accuracy and precision. Titrimetric analysis is based on the complete reaction between the analyte and a reagent, the *titrant*:

$$a\text{A} + t\text{T} \longrightarrow \text{products}$$

Where A and T represent the analyte and titrant, respectively and a and t are the stoichiometric coefficients. Titrations are often classified by the nature of this titration reaction: acid-base, redox, precipitation and complexation reactions are the most common reaction types.

Quantitative determination of the analyte concentration requires the following:

1. There is a stoichiometric reaction between the analyte and titrant. The reaction should be fast and complete, and the values of a and t must be known.

2. The concentration of the titrant solution must be known accurately.

3. The titrant solution must be *standardized* either by preparing it using a primary standard or more commonly, titrating it against a solution prepared with a primary standard.

4. The endpoint volume must be measured accurately using an appropriate chemical indicator or instrumental method.

5. If an instrumental method is used to follow the progress of the titration reaction, a titration curve may be generated, which allows for the analysis of mixtures and/or the detection of interferences.

Common Terms used in Titrimetric Analysis

Titration: It is the process of adding the solution (with known volume and concentration) from burette to the solution or analyte (known volume) whose concentration is to be determined until the reaction is just complete. It is also known as "titrimetric analysis"

Titrant: It is the solution of known concentration, whose fixed volume is added from burette to react with the analyte of unknown concentration.

Titrate: The active substance in solution to be determined by titration is called "titrate"

Equivalence point: It is the point (reading on burette) at which the reaction is just complete in a titration process and is also called as theoretical or stochiometric point.

End point: It is the point at which the indicator gives a visual color change and it is usually slightly higher than the equivalence point.

Indicators: An auxiliary reagent which is used to obtain the visual point at which titration is completed is called as "indicator". Usually, the smallest possible quantity of the indicator which can produce a visible color change is used.

There are three types of indicators which are in use:

Internal indicators: These are the substances which are to be added in the reacting medium to produce a change in color at the end point e.g., phenolphthalein or methyl orange in the titrations of acids and alkalies.

External indicators: Some indicators cannot be added in the reacting medium because of

1. If the indicator is a dark color liquid, the sudden change of color cannot be observed clearly

2. If the indicator forms an insoluble precipitate with the solution to which it has been added, in such a case the result will be low. In that case external indicators have to be used e.g., $K_3[Fe(CN)_6]$ is use as an external indicator in the titration of $K_2Cr_2O_7$ and ferrous ammonium sulphate in acid medium.

Self indicators: In the titration of oxalic acid and ferrous ammonium sulphate with $KMnO_4$ solution, as soon as the reaction is complete, and a drop of the $KMnO_4$ is in excess, a light pink color is itself developed, indicating that the reaction is complete and the end point has reached. Thus $KMnO_4$ here acts as a self indicator.

Mixed indicators: When a sharp color change is required over a narrow pH range, it is not easily attained by using ordinary acid-base indicators. For this purpose a suitable mixture of indicators is used. Indicators are selected and mixed in such a way that they have close pK_{In} values and the overlapping colors are complementary at an intermediate pH. A mixture of phenolphthalein (3 parts of 0.1 % solution in ethanol) and 1-naphthophthalein (1 part of 0.1% solution in ethanol) passes from pale yellow to rose color at pH 8.9. This mixed indicator is suitable for the titration of phosphoric acid to diprotic stage.

Primary standards: A primary standard is that which is sufficiently accurate and not needed to be calibrated by other standard rather used to calibrate other standards referred to as working standards. e.g., sodium carbonate, potassium hydrogen phthalate, potassium dichromate, oxalic acid are some of the primary standards. These are available in pure form and its solutions can be prepared by dissolving accurately weighed amount of these in water and making up the solutions to desired volume by addition of water. The essential features of a primary standard are:

1. It must be cheap and easy available
2. Low hygroscopicity
3. High equivalent weight
4. Low reactivity
5. High purity
6. Non toxic

Secondary standard: Often the titrant we use in a titration is not a primary standard, but is a second reagent which is prepared approximately to the correct concentration and then concentration is determined by comparing it with the primary standard. The second reagent is called a **secondary standard** and the process of calibrating the secondary standard against our primary standard is called **standardization**.

Glassware used in Laboratory

Pipette

There are three kinds of pipettes used in laboratory namely: transfer pipettes, graduated or measuring pipettes and syringe pipettes.

Transfer pipettes have one mark and deliver a constant volume of liquid under specified conditions. It consists of a long glass tube with large central cylindrical bulb; a calibration mark is etched around the upper (suction) tube and the lower (delivery) tube is drawn out to a fine tip (Figure 1.1). These pipettes are constructed with capacities of 1, 2, 5, 10, 20, 25, 50 and 100 mL.

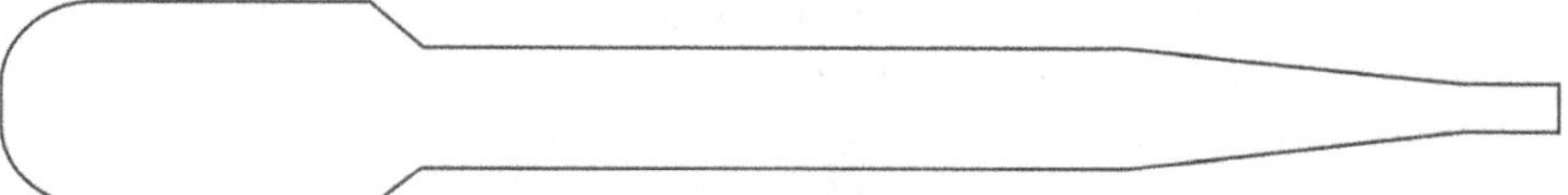

Fig. 1.1 Transfer pipette.

Graduated or measuring pipettes have graduated stems which are employed to deliver various small volumes as required (Figure 1.2). It consists of straight, fairly narrow tubes with no central bulb and is also constructed to a standard specification.

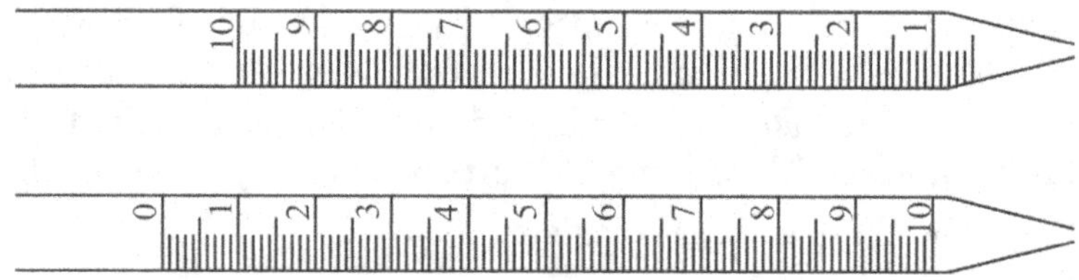

Fig. 1.2 Graduated pipette.

Syringe pipettes or micropipettes have fixed or variable volume and are usually employed for dispensing large numbers of identical volumes very quickly (Figure 1.3). These pipettes are now very common in laboratories and are used particularly for dispensing toxic solutions and large numbers of repeat volumes for multiple analysis. They may be of fixed or variable volumes. They have a push-button design in which the syringe is operated by pressing a button on the top of the pipette; the plunger travels between two fixed stops and a reliable constant volume of liquid is delivered. These pipettes are fitted with disposable plastic tips (usually of polythene or polypropylene) which are not wetted by aqueous solutions, thus helping to ensure constancy of the volume of liquid delivered. They are available in capacities of $1\,\mu L$ to 10 mL.

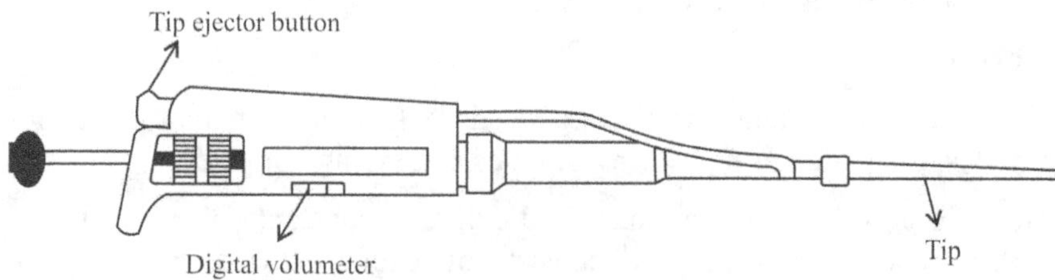

Fig. 1.3 Micropipette.

Note: The filling of pipettes should never be carried out by mouth suction and the pipette should never be placed to the lips, irrespective of which liquids are being measured.

Burettes

Burettes are long graduated cylindrical tubes of uniform bore terminating at the lower end in a glass or polytetrafluoroethylene (PTFE) stopcock and a jet. The PTFE taps have advantage that they do not require lubrication. A burette is employed with an extended jet which is bent at right angle so the tip of jet is displaced by few centimeters from the body of the burette. This would facilitate insertion of the tip of the burette into complicated glassware. If heated solutions have to be titrated, then the body of the burette should be kept away from the source of heat. Before using a burette it should be thoroughly cleaned by using a cleansing agent like chromic acid and then rinsing well with distilled water. After rinsing, the burette is clamped vertically using a clamp stand and then filled with required solution a little above the zero mark with the help of a funnel. The funnel is then removed and the liquid is discharged to the stopcock until the lower meniscus of the liquid is just below the zero mark. To read the position of the meniscus, eye must be at the same level as the meniscus to avoid any error (Figure 1.4).

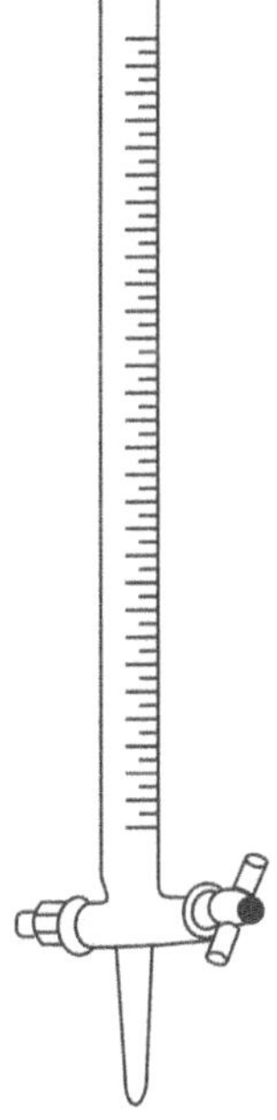

Fig. 1.4 Burette.

Graduated Flask

Graduated flask is also known as volumetric flask. It is a flat bottom, pear shaped flask with long narrow neck. A thin line is etched around the neck indicating the volume that a flask holds. The flask with one mark are always taken to contain a specified volume. It may also be marked to deliver a specified volume under certain condition. The mark extends completely around the neck in order to avoid any error. Graduated flask are available in a range of capacities of 1, 2, 5, 10, 50, 100, 200, 250, 500 2000 and 5000 mL. They are used in making a standard solution to a given volume and the solution can be obtained with the aid of pipettes (Figure 1.5).

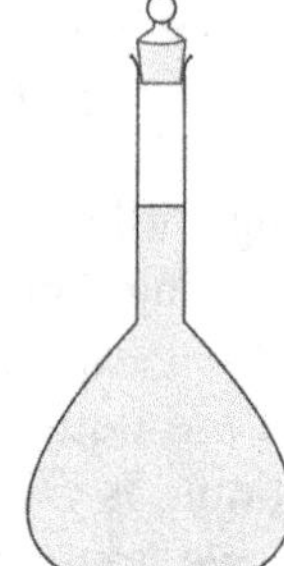

Fig.1.5 Graduated flask.

Graduated or Measuring Cylinders

These types of cylinders are available in capacities of 2 to 2000 mL. Since, the surface area of the liquid is much greater than in a graduated flask, the accuracy is not very high therefore it can only be used for rough measurements (Figure 1.6).

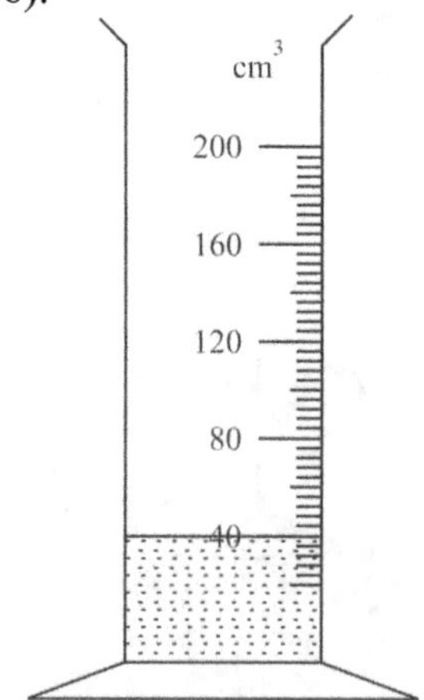

Fig. 1.6 Measuring cylinder.

Erlenmeyer Flask: (Conical Flask)

Erlenmeyer flask is also known as a conical flask. It is a widely used type of a laboratory flask which features a flat bottom; a conical body and a cylindrical neck. It is usually marked on the side to indicate the approximate volume of contents and has a spot of ground glass or enamel where it can be labeled with a pencil. It differs from the beaker in its tapered body and narrow neck. It is used in chemistry labs for titration e.g., for pH, as they can be held and the contents mixed single handed leaving the other hand free to add reagents. These type of flasks are suitable for heating liquids, e.g., with a Bunsen burner. The flask is usually placed on a ring held to a ring stand by means of a ring clamp. A wire gauze mesh or pad is usually placed between the rings and the flask to prevent the flames from directly touching the glass in the same manner as for a beaker. When heating (or cooling) in a water bath the flask can be clamped by the neck to a stand or a hooped weight may be placed over the conical part of the flask to prevent it from floating in the bath (Figure 1.7).

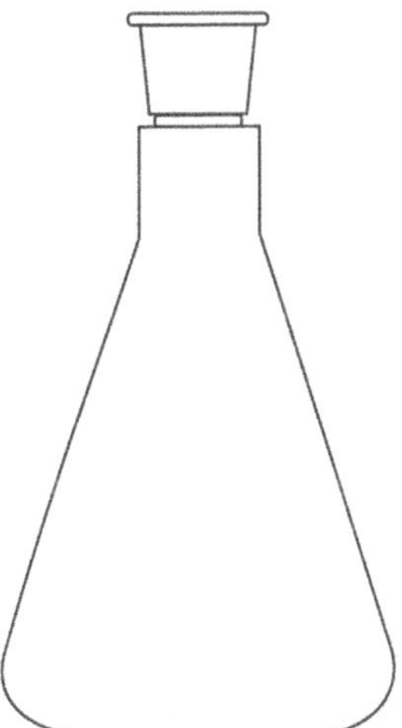

Fig. 1.7 Erlenmeyer flask.

Desiccator

A traditional desiccator is a glass bowl and lid each with thick glass rims that permit a seal when greased with a very thin film of Vaseline or a special grease in order to make it air tight (Figure 1.8). Desiccant (a hygroscopic chemical that absorbs water out of the air) is placed beneath the perforated ceramic disk. A sample in a beaker or crucible is placed on the top of this disk. The purpose of the desiccator is to either dry a chemical or keep a chemical from becoming "wet" from atmospheric humidity (water in the air). The drying agents (desiccants) used commonly are, anhydrous calcium chloride, silica gel, activated alumina and calcium sulphate anhydrous. It should be noted that the substance cannot be dried by the desiccant, whose vapour pressure is greater than that of the substance itself.

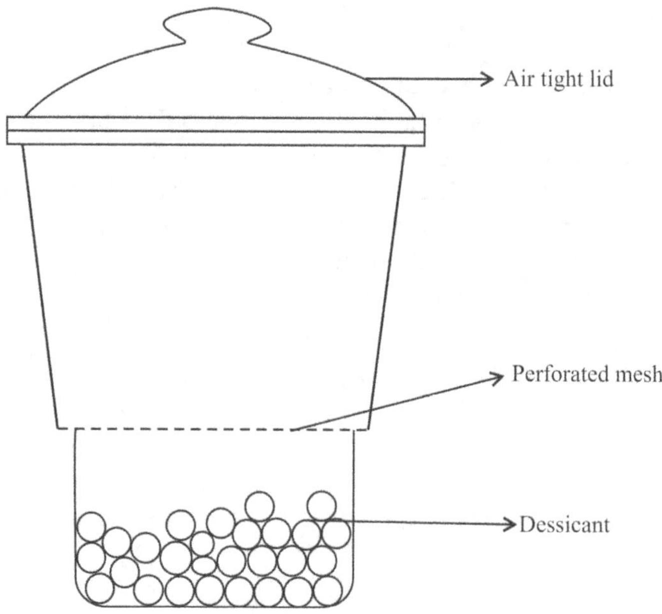

Fig. 1.8 Desiccator.

Calibration of Volumetric Glasswares

Volumetric glassware generally used is burettes, pipettes, volumetric flasks for measurement of accurate volume. Reliability of these volumetric glasswares depends upon the volume actually contained/delivered by that glassware. The calibration vertexes the volumes, which are actually contained or delivered and if it is lacking, it provide correction in the volume. The Indian standards Institution has specified 27 °C as the temperature at which glassware is calibrated. Since laboratory temperature is usually not exactly 27 °C glassware must be calibrated when used at other temperature. This is because of errors due to expansion (or contraction) of both glass vessel itself and solution contained there in. The coefficient of expansion of glass is sufficiently small and the correction required for this factor is negligible. The change in the volume of the solution itself is also important but it can still be ignored in many cases if working temperature is reasonably constant and is around 27 °C.

It may be noted that, the volumetric glassware should meet the standards laid down by the Indian Standard Institution (ISI) and such glasswares should be purchased in analytical laboratory. However, because of the high cost the certified glassware of ISI speccifications, less expensive are used after calibration.

Since most analytical work involves dilute aqueous solutions, distilled water is generally used as the reference material in the calibration of volumetric glassware. The general principle is to determine the weight of water into volume via. the density.

Calibration of Burette

A burette is a long calibrated glass tube with a fine end tip and a glass stopcock to allow controlled flow of volume. It affords greater precision, typically 0.1 to 0.2 %. Burette is principally used in titrations for the accurate delivery of a standard solution to the sample solution until the end point is reached. The conventional burettes for macro titrations are marked in 0.1 mL increments and are available in capacities of 10, 25, 50 and 100 mL micro-burettes are available in the capacities of down to 2 mL where the volume is marked in 0.01 mL increments.

Procedure for the Calibration of Burette
1. Fill the burette with distilled water and force any air bubbles out the tip. See whether the burette drains without leaving drops on its walls.
2. If drops are left, clean the burette with soap and water or soak it with cleaning solution.
3. Adjust the meniscus to be at or slightly below 0.00 mL, and touch the burette tip to a beaker to remove the suspended drop of water.
4. Allow the burette to stand for 5 min while weighing a 125-mL flask fitted with a rubber stopper.
5. If the level of the liquid in the burette has changed, tighten the stopcock and repeat the procedure. Record the level of the liquid.
6. Drain approximately 10 mL of water at a rate < 20 mL/min into the weighed flask and cap it tightly to prevent evaporation.

7. Allow 30 s for the film of liquid on the walls to descend before reading the burette. Estimate all readings to the nearest 0.01 mL. Weigh the flask again to determine the mass of water delivered.

8. Drain the burette from 10 to 20 mL and measure the mass of water delivered.

9. Repeat the procedure for 30, 40, and 50 mL. Then repeat the entire procedure (10, 20, 30, 40, 50 mL) a second time.

10. The difference between actual volume and apparent volume is the correction.

11. Calibration of burette is repeated as a check on work and duplicate results should agree within 0.04 mL.

Calibration of Pipette

The pipette is used to transfer a known volume of solution from one container to another. There are two common types of pipettes, the volumetric (transfer) pipette and measuring pipette. Volumetric pipette are used for high accuracy analytical work. They are calibrated to deliver a specified volume at a given temperature and are available in sizes from 0.5 to 200 mL. Measuring are straight bore pipette that are marked at 6 different volume intervals. They are convenient for delivering various volumes with reasonable 0.5 to 0.01 mL accuracy. They are not as accurate because of non uniformity of the internal diameter. Pipette must be calibrated if higher accuracy is required.

Procedure for the Calibration of Pipette

1. Weigh an Erlenmeyer flask to the nearest mg and record this value.

2. Record the temperature of the water. Carefully fill the pipette with water up to the graduated mark and deliver the water to the flask in the appropriate manner.

3. Stopper the container and reweigh it.

4. Use the difference in mass between each set of two consecutive mass measurements to determine the mass of water delivered in each trial (thus the origin of the name "weighing by difference").

5. Calculate the true volume as in the example for a 10 mL volumetric pipette that follows.

6. Duplicate calibrations should agree to within 0.01 mL.

7. Use the average value for all subsequent measurements with this pipette.

Calibration of Volumetric Flasks

Volumetric flasks are used in the preparation of standard solution and are available with capacities from 5 to 1000 mL. They are normally calibrated to contain a specific volume at 27 °C when filled to the line etched on the neck. Volumetric flask must thoroughly cleaned and rinsed with pure solvent before calibration.

Calibration of a volumetric flask is necessary only highest accuracy and it can be done by the following ways:

1. Volumetric flask is cleaned, rinsed and then clamped in an inverted position to dry it.

2. Stopper the flask and weigh to nearest milligram and record this weight.

3. Fill the flask with distilled water at room temperature. Adjust the lower meniscus of water to the etched level mark by means of pipette or dropper.

4. Stopper the flask and reweigh to the nearest milligram. Difference in weight gives the apparent volume of water contained and forms the weight of water, calculate the actual volume.

5. Calibration should be checked by repeating the procedure. Duplicate results should agree with in 0.3 mL for the flask.

Filtration

Filtration is commonly the mechanical or physical operation which is used for the separation of solids from fluids (liquids or gases) by interposing a medium through which only the fluid can pass. The success of filtration depends mostly on the fitting of the filter paper into the funnel. A funnel with an angle of 60 °C with a large stem is employed in order to get a quick filtration. The method for folding the filter paper has been shown in the Figure 1.9. For proper fitting into the funnel, the angle of the second fold should be adjusted until the filter paper fits well. If the filter paper is properly fitted, the stem of the funnel remains filled with the liquid throughout the filtration.

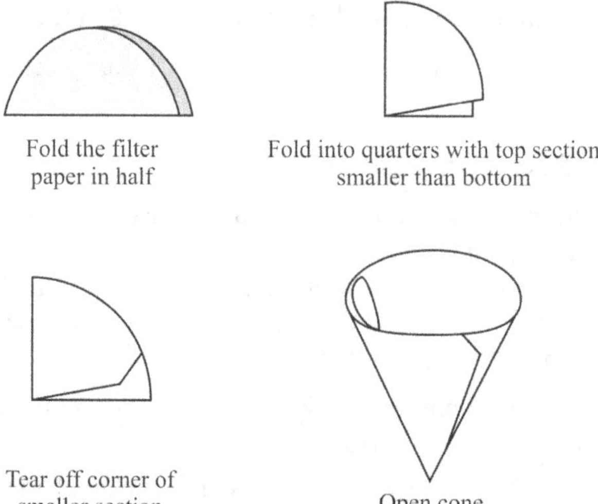

Fig. 1.9 Procedure for folding of filter paper.

The filter paper should never be completely filled with the solution and the level of the liquid must be about 1.5 cm below the upper edge of the filter paper. The process of correct filtration is shown in Figure 1.10.

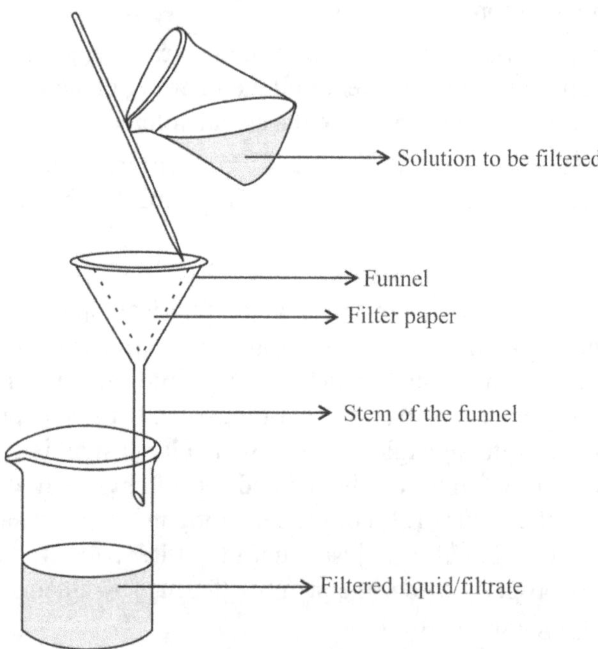

Fig. 1.10 Filtration method.

Sometimes in order to separate crystals from the mother liquor, the filtration is done using Buchner funnel i.e., a filtration flask attached to a vacuum pump. A circular filter paper of the size of bottom of the Buchner funnel is cut and fitted. It is wetted by means of liquid used for crystallization. The mixture to be filtered is poured slowly on the filter paper and suction is applied in order to drain out the solvent (Figure 1.11).

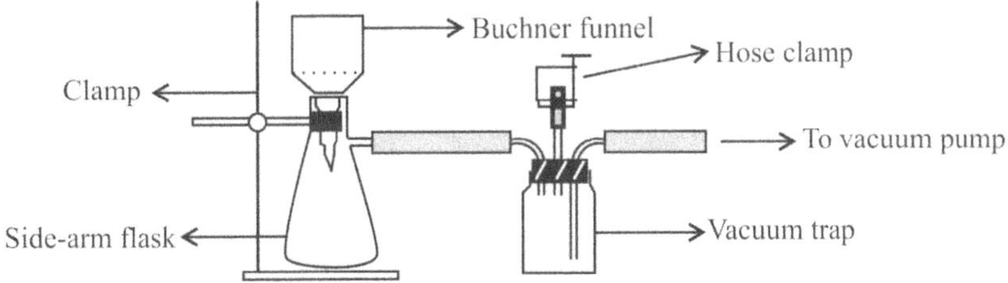

Fig. 1.11 Filtration using buchner funnel.

Analytical Balance

The important parts of the analytical balance are:

1. Supports
2. Pans
3. Plumb line
4. Beam
5. Pointer
6. Graduated scale
7. Knob (Arrest control)

The most important part of the analytical balance is beam which is an equal-armed lever furnished with long vertical pointer, by the deflection of which the movement of the beam can be judged. The lower end of the pointer swings in front of scale with divisions for reading the amplitude of swing. The scale has a zero line in the middle and 10 divisions on either side of it. When the beam is horizontal (the pans are balanced) the pointer should rest opposite the zero line of the scale.

The beam has agate knife-edges at its extremes, supporting stirrups from which balance pans are suspended. A steel knife edge is fixed exactly in the middle of the beam on its bottom side. This knife-edge faces downwards and supports the beam (Figure 1.12).

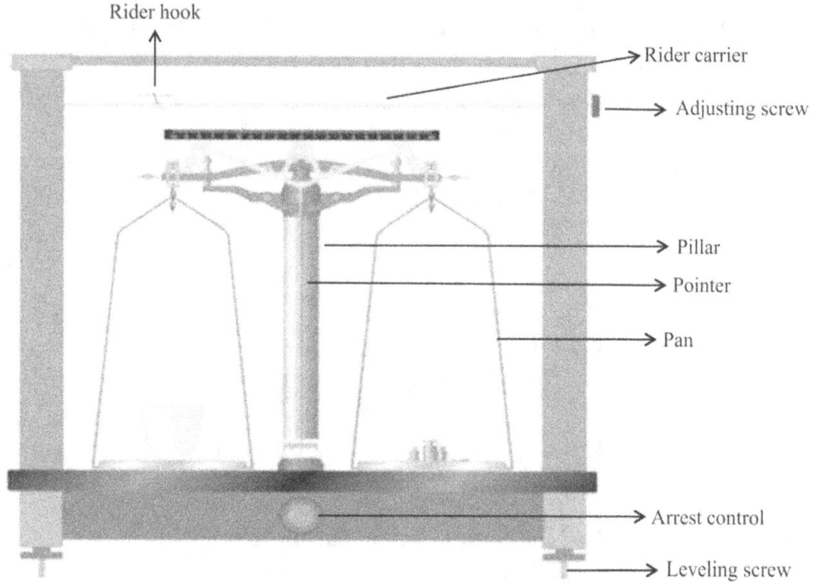

Fig. 1.12 Analytical balance.

Weight Box

The weights are made up of heavy metals alloy and are cylindrical in shape, each with a knob at the top. An ordinary set of weight contains 100 g, 50 g, 20 g, 10 g, 5 g, 2 g and 1 g weights. Weights smaller than 1 g are called as 'milligram' (mg) weights or fractional weights. They are leaf shaped foils of aluminum or other suitable metal with one of the sides turned up for picking up with forceps (Figure 1.13).

The fractional weights have 3 sets of 500 mg, 200 mg, 100 mg, 50 mg, 20 mg, 10 mg, 5 mg, 2 mg and 1 mg weights.

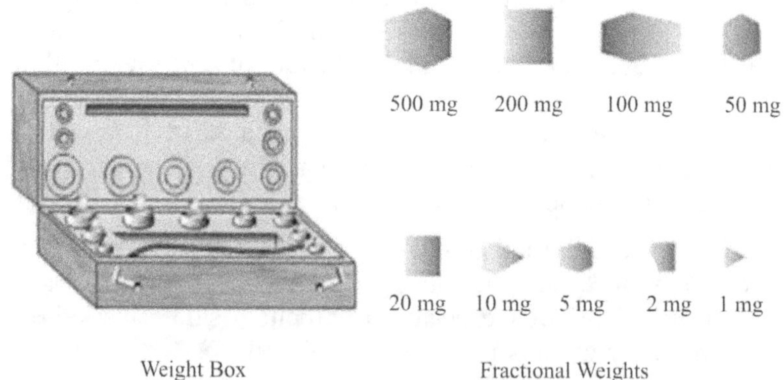

Fig. 1.13 Weight box and shape of fractional weights.

Rules in Weighing

To keep the balance in working order and to obtain accurate results the following rules should be observed:

1. Sit squarely in front of the balance while weighing.

2. Keep no objects inside the balance case except beakers with calcium chloride (to absorb moisture), which should be placed in the back corners of the case. Keep the balance clean. If anything gets spilled on the pan or the case bottom, sweep it out immediately with a soft brush.

3. Align the balance strictly vertical by its plumb line. Do not move the balance after alignment.

4. When weighing, open only the side doors of the case; do not raise its front door.

5. Never place the substance being weighed directly on the pan or on paper. Weigh solids on a watch glass or in a beaker and volatile and hygroscopic substances and liquids in weighing bottles. Glassware used for weighing should be clean and dry.

6. Objects being weighed should have the same temperature as the weighing room. To ensure this, keep them in a desiccator in the weighing room for at least 15 or 20 minutes before weighing.

7. Never load the balance above its maximum load (200 g).

8. Change the load on the balance only after fully arresting it.

9. Remove or add substance being weighed only outside the case.

10. During observation of pointer deflections, keep the case doors shut.

11. Never touch weights, pans, or balance beam. Handle weights only with plastic-tipped forceps.

12. Place weights on the right-hand pan, arranging them in the centre to avoid skewing of the pan, which may distort the reading.

13. Open the box of weights only when weighing.

14. Before and after using, keep the rider on the carrier hook clear of the beam scale.

15. After finishing weighing, move the carrier inside the case.

16. After weighing, arrest the balance and check record of the results. Without opening the case doors, remove the rider from the beam scale using the carrier rod, open the right-hand case door, replace the weights in their places in the box, open the left-hand case door, remove the object weighed from the scale pan and close the case door. After weighing, clean the balance with a brush or a piece of chamois leather to remove possible spillage or other dirt.

Calibration of Weights

The individual spent weights are calibrated against standards by the method of substitution to eliminate the possible error due to inequality of the length of the balance arms and are done as:

1. Place the standard weights on the left pan and adjust a tare on the right pan.

2. By the method of swings balance the weights exactly using a rider.

3. It is convenient to use the rider in the middle of the arm by placing extra 0.05 g weight on the left pan.

4. Now replace the standard weight by the weight to be calibrated and again determine the rest point.

5. Repeat this process for every piece in the weight box and determine a relation between the standard weight and the spent weight in the form of table showing the absolute error for each spent weight.

Electronic Balance

Electronic balance has many advantages like convenience in use, unaffected by mechanical failure and highly reduced sensitivity to vibration. With an electronic balance, operation of a single on-off control permits the operator to read the weight of an object on the balance pan immediately from a digital display. These types of balance can be coupled with a printer which gives a printed record of the weight. These balances also have a tare facility which permits the weight of a container to be cancelled out, so that when material is added to the container, the weight recorded is simply the weight of material used. The standard modern electronic balance is shown in Figure 1.14 below:

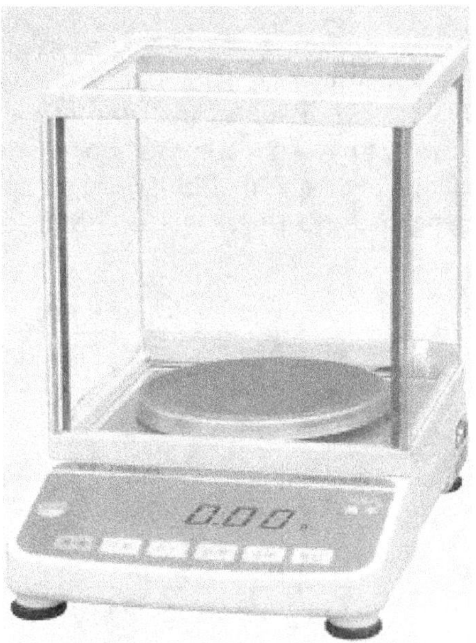

Fig. 1.14 Electronic balance.

Electronic balances are available in four weight ranges:

1. Up to about 200 g and reading to 0.1 mg (macrobalance)
2. Up to about 30 g and reading to 0.1 mg (semi-microbalance)
3. Up to about 20 g and reading to 1 μg (microbalance)
4. Up to about 5 g and reading to 0.1 μg (ultra-microbalance)

Standard Solution

The solution of an accurately known strength or concentration is called as a "standard solution". It contains a definite number of g equivalents/dm^3 (normal solution) or g moles/ dm^3 (molar solution) or g moles in 1 kg of solvent (molal solution) of the solute or substance.

Normal Solution

A normal solution is one which contains one g equivalent of the active reagent (equivalent weight in grams) dissolved in one dm^3 of the solution. Thus if 36.5 g of HCl are dissolved in 1 dm^3, this solution of HCl is 1 N. Therefore the normality is given as:

$$\text{Normality} = \frac{\text{no. of g equivalent of solute}}{\text{no. of liters (dm}^3) \text{ of solution}}$$

Molar Solution

A molar solution is one which contains one g mole of active reagent (molecular weight in grams) dissolved in 1 dm^3 of the solution. Thus if 36.5 g of HCl are dissolved in 1 dm^3, this solution of HCl is 1 M. In case of HCl, the equivalent weight and molecular weight are the same; hence the solution containing 36.5 g is 1 N as well as 1 M also. Thus molarity is given as:

$$\text{Molarity} = \frac{\text{no. of moles of solute}}{\text{no. of liters } (dm^3) \text{ of solution}}$$

Molal Solution

A molal solution is one which contains a known number of moles of the solute dissolved in 1 kg of the solvent.

$$\text{Molality} = \frac{\text{Moles of solute}}{\text{Mass of solvent in kg}}$$

Molarity varies with temperature because volume of solution varies with temperature where as molality is independent of temperature.

Problem: Determine the molarity and molality of a 17% solution (by weight) of H_2SO_4. Its density is 1.1000 g cm^{-3}. How much 100 cm^3 of this acid be diluted in order to prepare 1 N solution?

Solution: The H_2SO_4 solution is 17 %

Amount of H_2SO_4 present in 1000 g of solution = 170.0 g

And weight of water in 1000 g of solution = (1000 − 170) g = 830 g

$$\text{Amount of } H_2SO_4 \text{ present in 1000 g of water} = \frac{170 \times 1000}{830} g = 204.81g$$

$$\frac{204.81}{98} = 2.08 \text{ molal}$$

Hence molality is 2.08 molal

$$\text{Volume for 1000 g of solution is} = \frac{1000}{1.1} = 909.1 \text{ cm}^3$$

$$\text{Amount of } H_2SO_4 \text{ contained in 1 } dm^3 \text{ of solution} = \frac{170 \times 1000}{909.1} = 186.9 \text{ g}$$

Hence molarity of solution is 186.9/ 98 = 1.9 M

And Normality of this solution is $2 \times 1.9 = 3.8$ N

Let the new volume after dilution is V_1

So $1 \times V_1 = 100 \times 3.8$

$\qquad V_1 = 380 \text{ cm}^3$

Mole Fraction

It is defined as the ratio of the number of moles of solute to the total number of moles of the solution.

Mole fraction of a component

$$= \frac{\text{number of moles of the component}}{\text{Total number of moles of all the component in solution}}$$

Percentage Composition by Weight (weight percent)

It is defined as the number of grams of solute per 100 grams of solution. It can be expressed as:

$$P = \frac{W}{W + W_o} \times 100$$

Where P = % by weight of solute

$\qquad W$ = number of grams of solute

$\qquad W_o$ = number of grams of solvent

Percentage composition by volume (volume percent): The concentration is expressed in terms of the volume of the solute and solvent. For example, a 20% ethanol solution is prepared by adding 20 cm^3 of alcohol in 80 cm^3 of water.

Percentage Strength

10% of NaOH indicates 10 g of NaOH is present in 100 cm^3 of the solution and 10% H_2SO_4 means 10 g of H_2SO_4 in 100 cm^3 of the solution.

CHAPTER 1

Acids and Bases

Acids and Bases

First definition of acid was given by Svante Arrhenius (Sweden) in 1884, which states that an acid is a substance that can release a proton or hydrogen ion (H^+). Hydrogen chloride (HCl) in water solution ionizes and becomes hydrogen ions and chloride ions. The acids HCl, HNO_3, H_3PO_3, H_2SO_4, HBr, HI and HCN dissociate completely in water and thus are *strong acids*. A base or alkali, is a substance that can donate a hydroxide ion (OH^-). Sodium hydroxide (NaOH) in water solution becomes sodium ions and hydroxide ions. Bases like, NaOH, KOH, LiOH, $Sr(OH)_2$, $Ba(OH)_2$ and $Ca(OH)_2$ completely dissociates in water and are thus *strong bases*.

Three models of acids and bases

1. **Arrhenius model**

   Basis for the model-action in water

   - Acid definition: produces H^+ (hydrogen ion) in water solution
   - Base definition: produces OH^- (hydroxide ion) in water solution

2. **Bronsted-lowry model**

   Basis for the model-proton transfer

   - Acid definition: donates a proton
   - Base definition: accepts a proton
   - Conjugate acid definition: the acid becomes the conjugate base after it donates the proton because it can now accept it back.
   - Conjugate base definition: the base becomes the conjugate acid after it accepts the proton because it can now donate it back.

3. **Lewis model**

   Basis for model-electron pair transfer

   - Acid definition: accepts a pair of electrons
   - Base definition: donates a pair of electrons

Acid-Base Titration

Acid-base titration is a neutralization titration in which, titration of alkaline solution is carried out with a standard acid solution in order to determine the amount of acid which is exactly equivalent to the amount of base present. The point at which this is reached, is called **theoretical end point** and at this point whole acid reacts with base to form the corresponding salt. For any titration the correct end point will be characterized by a definite value of pH of the solution, which depends on the nature of acid, nature of the base and the concentration of the solution. A large number of substances, acid-base indicators, change the color of the solution according to the concentration of hydrogen ions present. Change in color from acid to alkaline or vice-versa is not sudden but takes place within a small interval of pH and is called **color change interval** of indicator. A list of indicators commonly used in acid-base titration is given in **Table 1.** For most acid-base titrations, an indicator that exhibits sharp color change at the pH close to the equivalent pH, is chosen.

Table 1 Common indicators used in acid-base titrations

Indicator	Color change pH interval	Acid color	Base Color
m-Cresol purple	0.5-2.5	Red	Yellow
Thymol Blue	1.2-2.8	Red	Yellow
Bromophenol blue	3.0-4.6	Yellow	Blue
Methyl orange	3.1-4.4	Red	Yellow
Methyl red	4.2-6.2	Red	Yellow
Phenol red	6.8-8.4	Yellow	Red
Thymol blue	8.0-9.6	Yellow	Blue
Phenolphthalein	8.2-10	Colorless	Red

EXPERIMENT 1.1

To Prepare 1M HCl and Standardize it and Perform Assay of Sodium Hydrogen Carbonate

Theory

Sodium hydrogen carbonate is a white crystalline or amorphous powder and saline in taste. It is freely soluble in water but practically insoluble in alcohol. It is used for its acid neutralizing properties. It is used as an antacid to treat heartburn, indigestion and other stomach disorders. Its aqueous solution is used as local applicant for burns, insect bites etc.

Sodium hydrogen carbonate is a base and it is titrated with dilute hydrochloric acid using methyl orange as indicator (pH: 3.1-4.4) and the equivalence point of the reaction is at 3.6 approximately.

Chemical reaction

$$Na_2CO_3 + HCl \longrightarrow NaHCO_3 + NaCl$$

$$NaHCO_3 + HCl \longrightarrow NaCl + CO_2 + H_2O$$

Chemicals required

1. 1.0 M HCl solution. Fill the volumetric flask up to 3/4th with distilled water. Add 85 ml of concentrated hydrochloric acid. Stopper the volumetric flask and shake the solution. Fill the volumetric flask with distilled water up to 1000 ml mark.

   Note: When diluting concentrated hydrochloric acid, remember to add concentrated acid (HCl) to water (and not water to HCl) in order to avoid spattering. Handle the containers carefully as dilution involves generation of heat.

2. Methyl orange as indicator
3. Anhydrous Sodium hydrogen carbonate

Procedure

1. Standardization of HCl

(i)   Weigh accurately 1.5g of anhydrous sodium carbonate and transfer it to conical flask.

(ii)   Dissolve it in 100mL of distilled water.

(iii)   Now add 0.1mL of methyl red indicator.

(iv)   Take 1.0 M HCl in a burette and fill the burette up to mark.

(v)   Add the acid slowly from the burette to the conical flask containing sodium carbonate solution.

(vi)   Keep on adding 1.0 M HCl with constant shaking until the appearance of faint pink color.

(vii)   Heat the solution, cool and continue titration.

(viii)   Repeat step vi and vii until the faint pink color is no longer affected by continuous heating.

2. Determination of percent purity of Sodium Hydrogen Carbonate

(i)   Weigh accurately 1.5 g of sodium hydrogen carbonate and transfer it to conical flask.

(ii)   Add 50 mL of distilled water to the conical flask to dissolve sodium hydrogen carbonate.

(iii)   Fill the burette with standardized 1.0 M HCl up to the mark.

(iv)   Add 0.2 mL methyl orange as an indicator.

(v)   Titrate the solution in the conical flask with standardized 1.0 M HCl.

(vi)   Stir the solution continuously until the appearance of end point i.e. color of the solution changes from orange to pink color.

Observation and Calculations

1. Standardization of HCl

The molarity of HCl is obtained by using the following relation:

$$\text{Molarity of HCl} = \frac{\text{moles of HCl}}{\text{liter}} = \frac{\text{moles of Na}_2\text{CO}_3 \times 2}{(\text{ml HCl}/1000)}$$

$$\text{Molarity of HCl} = \frac{\text{wt. of Na}_2\text{CO}_3 \times 2}{\text{mol. wt. of Na}_2\text{CO}_3 \times \text{volume of HCl (liter)}}$$

2. Percentage purity of $NaHCO_3$

Percentage purity

$$= \frac{\text{Burette reading} \times 0.084 \times \text{Molarity (calculated)} \times 100}{\text{Weight of sample} \times 1.0 \text{ (molarity known)}}$$

EXPERIMENT 1.2

To Prepare and Standardize 0.1 M NaOH and Perform the Assay of Boric Acid

Theory

Boric acid is a solid which is available in three forms: colorless, odorless pearly scales; six-sided triclinic crystals and white odorless powder. Boric acid is a local anti-infective and is used in dusting powders, local antiseptic creams, ointments, lotions and is applied on skin, eyes and mucous membrane. Aqueous solution of boric acid have been used as mouth washes and eye lotions as it possess weak bactericide and fungicide properties.

In this titration weak boric acid acts as a strong acid in the presence of glycerin due to the formation of Glyceroboric acid complex. This aids its titration with strong alkali, sodium hydroxide. Phenolphthalein is used as an indicator.

Chemical reaction

Glycerol $+$ H_3BO_3 $\longrightarrow$ Glyceroboric acid complex $+$ H_3O^+ $+$ H_2O

Glyceroboric acid complex $+$ NaOH $\longrightarrow$ Glycerol $+$ $NaBO_2$ (Sodium metaborate)

Chemicals required
1. 0.1 M sodium hydroxide solution
2. Boric acid
3. Potassium hydrogen phthalate
4. Glycerin
5. Phenolphthalein indicator

Procedure

1. Standardization of sodium hydroxide

(i) Weigh accurately 0.2 g of potassium hydrogen phthalate and transfer it to the conical flask.

(ii) Dissolve it in about 100 mL of water.

(iii) Add 0.1 ml of phenolphthalein as indicator.

(iv) Fill the burette up to mark with sodium hydroxide solution.

(v) Titrate potassium hydrogen phthalate by slowly adding sodium hydroxide solution from burette.

(vi) Continue the titration with continuous shaking until the appearance of light pink color persists for 30 secs.

(vii) Note the reading and again perform the experiment for two more times.

(viii) Take three concordant reading and calculate the morality of given sample of sodium hydroxide.

2. Assay of boric acid

(i) Take 25mL of glycerin in conical flask.

(ii) Add 2 drops of phenolphthalein in it.

(iii) Neutralize the solution by titrating with standardized sodium hydroxide solution.

(iv) Continue the titration till light pink color is obtained.

(v) Now add 50 mL of water in it.

(vi) Take 0.5 mg boric acid in another conical flask.

(vii) Add the above solution in it.

(viii) Shake the solution and add 1 drop of phenolphthalein in it.

(ix) Titrate it with sodium hydroxide by slowly adding the solution from burette.

(x) Continue the titration till permanent pink color is obtained.

(xi) Take the reading by performing the experiment three times.

(xii) Calculate the percentage purity.

Observation and Calculation

Determination of molarity of NaOH

Molarity of NaOH

$$= \frac{\text{Weight of potassium hydrogen phthalate}}{\text{Mol. wt. of pot. hydrogen phthalate} \times \text{volume of NaOH (liter)}}$$

EXPERIMENT 1.3

To Prepare and Standardize 0.1 M NaOH and Perform Assay of Ammonium Chloride

Theory

In this titration aqueous solution of ammonium chloride is first treated with formaldehyde which results in the liberation of hydrochloric acid equivalent to the amount of ammonium chloride present in the solution. This hydrochloric in turn reacts with sodium hydroxide.

Chemical equation

$$4NH_4Cl \; + \; 4H_2O \longrightarrow 4NH_4OH \; + \; 4HCl$$

Ammonium
Chloride

Ammonium
hydroxide

$$4NH_4OH \; + \; 6HCHO \longrightarrow (CH_2)_6N_4 \; + \; 10\,H_2O$$

Formaldehyde

Hexamine

$$4\,HCl \; + \; 4NaOH \longrightarrow 4NaCl \; + \; 4H_2O$$

Sodium
hydroxide

Chemicals required

0.1 M sodium hydroxide solution

Potassium hydrogen phthalate

Phenolphthalein indicator

Procedure

Standardization of sodium hydroxide

- (i) Weigh accurately 0.2 g of potassium hydrogen phthalate and transfer it to the conical flask.
- (ii) Dissolve it in about 100 mL of water.
- (iii) Add 0.1mL of phenolphthalein indicator.
- (iv) Fill the burette up to mark with sodium hydroxide solution.
- (v) Titrate the above solution by slowly adding sodium hydroxide solution from the burette.
- (vi) Continue the titration with continuous shaking until the appearance light pink color persists for 30 secs.
- (vii) Note the reading and again perform the experiment for two more times.
- (viii) Take three concordant reading and calculate the morality of given sample of sodium hydroxide.

Determination of ammonium chloride

- (i) Weigh accurately about 0.1 g ammonium chloride and transfer it to conical flask.
- (ii) Dissolve it in 20 mL of distilled water.
- (iii) Add a mixture of 5 mL formaldehyde, 0.1 mL phenolphthalein and 20 mL of distilled water.
- (iv) Fill the burette with standardized 0.1 M NaOH solution.
- (v) Titrate the solution with 0.1 M NaOH using further 0.2 mL phenolphthalein as indicator.

Observations and Calculations

Standardization of sodium hydroxide

Molarity of NaOH

$$= \frac{\text{Weight of potassium hydrogen phthalate}}{\text{Mol. wt. of pot. hydrogen phthalate} \times \text{volume of NaOH (liter)}}$$

Assay of ammonium chloride

Molarity of NaOH

$$= \frac{\text{Volume of NaOH used (ml)} \times \text{molarity (cal)} \times 100}{\text{Weight of sample} \times \text{molarity (given)}}$$

EXPERIMENT 1.4

To Prepare and Standardize 0.5 M H_2SO_4 and Perform Assay of Sodium Carbonate

Theory

It is having not less than 99.0 % and not more than 105.0 % of sodium carbonate. It is used as an antacid and topically as lotion in dermatitis. Sodium carbonate being basic in nature is titrated with dilute sulphuric acid using bromophenol blue indicator. Due to the formation of carbonic acid during the titration, pH of the solution becomes acidic. Thus, bromophenol blue is an indicator of choice (pH range, 3.6-4.4).

Chemical equation

$$Na_2CO_3 + H_2SO_4 \longrightarrow Na_2SO_4 + H_2O + CO_2$$

Chemicals required

0.5 M H_2SO_4 solution. Pour 15 mL of H_2SO_4 in 400 mL of distilled water in a 500 mL volumetric flask. Shake the solution and adjust the volume up to 500 mL mark with distilled water.

Bromophenol blue indicator

Anhydrous sodium carbonate

Methyl orange indicator

Procedure

Standardization of H_2SO_4

(i)   Weigh accurately about 0.3 g of anhydrous sodium carbonate.

(ii)   Transfer the weighed sodium carbonate to a conical flask and add 100 mL of distilled water and dissolve it completely.

(iii)   Add 2-3 drops of methyl orange indicator.

(iv)   Add 0.5M H_2SO_4 into the burette and fill it up to mark.

(v)   Titrate the solution in conical flask with 0.5M H_2SO_4 until the color of solution changes from yellow to orange.

(vi) Take three concordant readings and calculate the molarity of H_2SO_4.

(vii) Each ml of 0.5M H_2SO_4 solution = 0.05299 g or 52.99 mg of sodium carbonate.

Assay of sodium carbonate

(i)   Weigh accurately about 0.5 g of sodium carbonate and transfer it to the conical flask.

(ii) Dissolve it in 20 mL of water.

(iii) Titrate the solution with 0.5M H_2SO_4 slowly by adding the solution drop wise to the conical flask.

(iv) Bromophenol blue is used as an indicator.

(v)   Continue titration until the color changes from blue to yellow at end point.

Observation and Calculations

Standardization of H_2SO_4

Molarity of H_2SO_4 =

$$\frac{\text{Weight of sod. carbonate (g)}}{\text{Mol. wt. of sod. carbonate} \times \text{vol. of } H_2SO_4 \text{ consumed (liter)}}$$

Assay of sodium carbonate

$$\text{Percentage purity} = \frac{\text{Volume of } H_2SO_4 \text{ used (mL)} \times \text{molarity (cal)} \times 100}{\text{Weight of sample} \times \text{molarity (given)}}$$

EXPERIMENT 1.5

To Determine Percentage Purity of Zinc Oxide

Theory

It does not have more than 99.0% of zinc oxide which has been calculated with reference of the substance which is ignited to constant weight. Zinc oxide occurs as a soft, white, fine powder, free from grittiness. it is used as a mild antiseptic and astringent. It is assistive in the treatment of eczema, ringworm, varicose ulcers and psoriasis.

Assay of zinc oxide is a type of back titration because its reaction with sulphuric acid is slow. Excess of sulphuric acid is added to the reaction mixture and excess of acid is back titrated with sodium hydroxide.

Chemical equation

$$ZnO + H_2SO_4 \longrightarrow ZnSO_4 + H_2O$$

$$H_2SO_4 + 2\ NaOH \longrightarrow Na_2SO_4 + 2H_2O$$

Chemicals required

0.5M H_2SO_4 solution: Pour 15 mL of H_2SO_4 in 400 mL of distilled water in a 500 mL volumetric flask. Shake the solution and adjust the volume up to 500 mL mark with distilled water.

0.5 M NaOH solution.

Methyl red indicator.

Procedure

Standardization of H_2SO_4

   (i)   Weigh accurately about 0.3 g of anhydrous sodium carbonate.

   (ii)   Transfer the weighed sodium carbonate to a conical flask and add 100 ml of distilled water and dissolve it completely.

(iii)   Add 2-3 drops of methyl orange indicator.

(iv)   Titrate the solution with 0.5M H_2SO_4 by slowly adding the solution from burette.

(v)   Continue titration until the color of solution changes from yellow to orange.

(vi)   Take three concordant readings and calculate the molarity of H_2SO_4.

(vii)   Each ml of 0.5M H_2SO_4 solution = 0.05299 g or 52.99 mg of sodium carbonate.

Determination of zinc oxide

(i)   Weigh accurately about 1.5 g of zinc oxide and 2.5 g of ammonium chloride.

(ii)   Transfer the weighed substance to the conical flask.

(iii)   Dissolve them in 50 mL of 0.5 mL sulphuric acid by gentle heating.

(iv)   Add few drops of methyl red indicator

(v)   Titrate the solution with 0.5M NaOH solution until yellow color appears at the end point.

Observation and Calculations

Standardization of H_2SO_4

Molarity of H_2SO_4 =

$$\frac{\text{Weight of sod. carbonate (g)}}{\text{Mol. wt. of sod. carbonate} \times \text{vol. of } H_2SO_4 \text{ consumed (liter)}}$$

Assay of zinc oxide

Molecular weight of zinc oxide = 81.41

Weight of sample = W g

Volume of 0.5M NaOH consumed by unreacted sulphuric acid = M mL

If the molarity of sodium hydroxide and sulphric acid is same

Volume of 0.5M sulphuric acid reacted with zinc oxide = 50 – M = V mL

From equation

1 mole of ZnO = 1 mole of H_2SO_4 = 1000 mL of 1M H_2SO_4 solution

Each mL of 0.5M H_2SO_4 = 0.04068 g of ZnO

$$\text{Percentage purity} = \frac{0.04068 \times V \times \text{molarity (cal)} \times 100}{W \times \text{molarity (known)}}$$

EXPERIMENT 1.6

To Determine Percentage Purity of Sodium Phosphate

Theory

Sodium phosphate is dodecahydrate of disodium hydrogen orthophosphate. It contains not less than 98.5 % and not more than 101.0 % sodium phosphate. It occurs in the form of colorless transparent crystals, with a saline taste. It is used as saline laxative, cathartic and buffering agent.

In this titration basic sodium phosphate reacts with hydrochloric acid to form sodium dihydrogen phosphate in the presence of bromocresol green indicator.

Chemical equation

$$Na_2HPO_4 \ + \ HCl \ \longrightarrow \ NaH_2PO_4 \ + \ NaCl$$

Sodium phosphate   Sodium dihydrogen phosphate

Chemicals required

1. 0.5M HCl solution. To prepare this solution add 45 mL of concentrated HCl solution into water and make up the volume to 1 liter.

2. Bromocresol green.

3. Sodium phosphate

Procedure

1. **Standardization of 0.5M HCl solution**

   (i) Weigh accurately 1.2 g of anhydrous sodium carbonate and transfer it to the volumetric flask containing 100 mL of distilled water.

   (ii) Dissolve sodium carbonate completely and make up the volume of solution up to 250 mL with distilled water.

(iii) Take 25 mL of this solution in a conical flask and add 2-3 drops of methyl orange indicator.

(iv) Fill the burette with hydrochloric acid solution and make it up to mark.

(v) Titrate the solution with given hydrochloric acid solution until the color changes from yellow to orange at the end point.

(vi) Take three concordant readings and calculate the molarity of hydrochloric acid.

2. Assay of sodium phosphate

(i) Weigh accurately 1.5 g of sodium phosphate

(ii) Transfer the weighed sodium phosphate to the conical flask and dissolve it in 100 mL of distilled water.

(iii) Add a few drops of bromocresol green indicator to the above solution.

(iv) Fill the burette up to mark with standardized hydrochloric acid.

(v) Titrate the solution in the conical flask with standardized hydrochloric acid by adding the solution drop wise from the burette.

(vi) Continue the titration until the appearance of green color at the end point.

Observation and Calculations

1 mole of sodium phosphate = 1 mole of HCl = 1000 ml of 1M HCl solution

Each ml of 0.5M HCl solution = 0.01791 g of sodium phosphate

% purity of sodium phosphate =

$$\frac{0.01791 \times \text{vol.of HCl used (ml)} \times \text{molarity (cal)} \times 100}{\text{Weight of the sample} \times \text{molarity (known)}}$$

EXPERIMENT 1.7

To Determine Percentage Purity of Sodium Benzoate

Theory

Sodium benzoate is sodium salt of benzoic acid which is derived from a reaction of benzoic acid with sodium hydroxide. It is used as a preservative in carbonated drinks, jams, fruit juices, pickles and condiments. Sodium benzoate liberates sodium hydroxide which in turn reacts with hydrochloric acid. Reaction is carried out using bromophenol blue as indicator and ether is added to dissolve benzoic acid formed in the reaction.

Chemical equation

$$C_6H_5COONa \ + \ HCl \ \longrightarrow \ C_6H_5COOH \ + \ NaCl$$

Chemicals required

1. 0.5M *HCl solution*: To prepare this solution add 45 mL of concentrated HCl solution into water and make up the volume to 1 liter.
2. Bromophenol blue indicator.
3. Ether.

Procedure

1. **Standardization of 0.5M HCl solution**

   (i)   Weigh accurately 1.2 g of anhydrous sodium carbonate and transfer it to the volumetric flask containing 100 mL of distilled water.

   (ii) Dissolve sodium carbonate completely and make up the volume of the solution up to 250 mL with distilled water.

   (iii) Take 25 mL of this solution in a conical flask and add 2-3 drops of methyl orange indicator.

   (iv) Fill the burette with given hydrochloric acid solution.

(v)   Titrate the solution in the conical flask with hydrochloric acid by adding the solution drop wise from the burette.

(vi)   Continue titration until the color changes from yellow to orange at the end point.

(vii)   Take three concordant readings and calculate molarity of hydrochloric acid.

2. Assay of sodium phosphate

(i)   Weigh accurately 1.5 g of sodium benzoate and transfer it to a 250 mL stoppered-conical flask.

(ii)   Dissolve it in 25 mL of distilled water and add 75 mL of ether.

(iii)   Add 2-3 drops of bromophenol blue indicator.

(iv)   Fill the burette with standardized 0.5M hydrochloric acid solution.

(v)   Titrate the solution with 0.5M hydrochloric acid with continuous shaking in order to mix water and ether layer.

(vi)   Continue titration until light green color persists in the water layer.

Observation and Calculations

Assay of sodium benzoate

1 mole of sodium benzoate = 1 mole of HCl = 1000 mL of 1M HCl solution

Each ml of 0.5M HCl solution = 0.07205 g of sodium benzoate

% purity

$$= \frac{0.07205 \times \text{vol.of } 0.5M \text{ HCl used (mL)} \times \text{molarity (cal)} \times 100}{\text{Weight of sodium benzoate used} \times \text{molarity (known)}}$$

EXPERIMENT 1.8

Determination of Percent Purity of Sodium Potassium Tartrate

Theory

Sodium potassium tartrate is a double salt and is popularly called Rochelle salt. It has been used medicinally as a laxative. It is also used in silvering of mirrors. It is an ingredient of Fehling solution. In this experiment, sodium potassium tartrate is ignited and salt gets converted to respective carbonates (sodium carbonate and potassium carbonate) equivalent to the amount of salt. If the salt is heated strongly, alkali carbonates may be converted to respective oxides. These carbonates formed are basic in nature and reacts with sulphuric acid during the titration. It is a type of back titration and the excess of acid is titrated with sodium hydroxide.

Chemical equation

$$2\ C_4H_4O_6\ NaK\ .\ 4H_2O \longrightarrow Na_2CO_3\ +\ K_2CO_3$$

Chemicals required

1. Sodium potassium tartrate.
2. Methyl red-methylene blue TS
3. 0.5N NaOH

Procedure

1. **Standardization of 0.5N sodium hydroxide**
    (i)   Weigh accurately 0.2 g of potassium hydrogen phthalate.
    (ii) Transfer the weighed potassium hydrogen phthalate to the conical flask and dissolve it in about 100 mL of water.
    (iii) Add 0.1mL of phenolphthalein indicator.
    (iv) Fill the burette up to mark with given sodium hydroxide solution.

(v) Titrate the solution in conical flask with given sodium hydroxide solution by adding the solution drop wise.

(vi) Continue the titration with continuous shaking until the light pink color persists for 30 sec.

(vii) Note the reading and again perform the experiment twice.

(viii) Take three concordant reading and calculate the morality of given sample of sodium hydroxide.

2. **Assay of sodium potassium tartrate**

(i) Weigh accurately 2 g of sodium potassium tartrate and transfer it to a dry crucible.

(ii) Gently ignite the crucible in order to carbonize the salt thoroughly.

(iii) Cool the crucible and place it in a glass beaker.

(iv) Transfer the carbonized mass to the glass beaker with glass rod.

(v) Add 50 mL of water and 50 mL 0.5N sulphuric acid solution.

(vi) Boil the solution for 30 min.

(vii) Filter the solution and wash with water until it is neutral to litmus.

(viii) Cool the combined filtrate, add methyl red-methylene blue TS as indicator.

(ix) Titrate the above solution by slowly adding 0.5M sodium hydroxide solution from the burette.

Observation and Calculations

$$\% \text{ purity of sod. Pot. Tartrate} = \frac{a - b \times \text{eq. wt.} \times 100}{\text{Sample weight}}$$

a = amount of sulphuric acid used

b = amount of NaOH used in back titration

EXPERIMENT 1.9

To Determine Aspirin Content in Tablet Formulation

Theory

Aspirin belongs to a group of drugs called salicylates. It inhibits the synthesis of substances (prostaglandins) in the body which are responsible for pain, fever, and inflammation. Aspirin is used to treat mild to moderate pain, and also to reduce fever or inflammation. It is sometimes used to treat or prevent heart attacks, strokes and angina. Aspirin is a weak acid that undergoes slow hydrolysis; i.e., each aspirin molecules react with two hydroxide ions. To overcome this problem, a known excess amount of base is added to the sample solution and HCl titration is carried out to determine the amount of unreacted base. This is subtracted from the initial amount of base to find the amount of base that is actually reacted with the aspirin and hence the quantity of aspirin in the analyte.

Chemical equation

Aspirin $+ OH^-$ $\xrightarrow{\text{Fast}}$ $+ H_2O$

Aspirin $+ OH^-$ $\xrightarrow{\text{Slow}}$ $+ CH_3COO^-$

Chemicals required

1. 0.1M HCl solution. Add 8.5 mL of HCl solution to 100 mL of water. Make up the volume to 1 liter with water.
2. 0.1M NaOH solution. Dissolve 4.2 g of NaOH in 1000 mL of water.
3. Aspirin.
4. Phenolphthalein indicator.
5. Phenol red indicator.

Procedure

1. Weigh accurately 20 tablets and calculate the average weight of tablets.
2. Powder the tablets.
3. Accur weigh powder equivalent to 0.5 g of aspirin.
4. Dissolve in 10 to 15 mL alcohol and add 4 drops of phenolphthalein indicator.
5. Titrate each sample quickly to the first persistent faint pink color with standard 0.1M NaOH solution.
6. Record this volume.
7. Then add, same volume again +5 mL excess from the burrette.
8. Place the flasks on the steam bath for 45 minutes to allow reaction to proceed to completion.
9. Then back-titrate the excess base with your standard 0.1M HCl solution using phenol red as indicator.

Observation and Calculations

1. Determination of aspirin content in tablet

Volume of 0.1M NaOH added = 50 mL.

Moles of NaOH = $0.050 \times 0.10 = 5.0 \times 10^{-3}$.

Suppose, volume of 0.1M HCl required to react with excess of unreacted 0.1M NaOH solution is 30 mL.

Moles of HCl = Moles of excess of NaOH = $0.030 \times 0.10 = 3.0 \times 10^{-3}$

Moles of NaOH which reacted with aspirin:

$$5.0 \times 10^{-3} - 3.0 \times 10^{-3} = 2.0 \times 10^{-3} \text{ or } \frac{2.0 \times 10^{-2}}{2} \text{ moles of aspirin}$$

Mass of aspirin = $1.0 \times 10^{-3} \times 180 = 0.180$ g of aspirin

CHAPTER 2

Oxidation Reduction Titrations

Oxidation Reduction Titrations

These titrations are also known as redox titrations. This type of titrations are based on redox reaction (i.e., oxidation and reduction occurs simultaneously) between analyte and titrant. Redox titrations may involve use of redox indicators. Redox reaction may be referred as electron transfer reactions. A good example of redox reaction is the reaction between hydrogen and fluorine in which hydrogen is being oxidized and fluorine is being reduced.

The oxidation reaction is $H_2 + F_2 \longrightarrow 2HF$

And the reduction reaction is $H_2 \longrightarrow 2H^+ + 2e^-$

In oxidation reaction, the hydrogen is oxidized from an oxidation state of zero to an oxidation state of +1 and in reduction reaction; fluorine is reduced from an oxidation state of zero to an oxidation state of -1. When adding the reaction together the electrons are cancelled.

$$H_2 \longrightarrow 2H^+ + 2e^-$$

$$F_2 + 2e \longrightarrow 2F$$

$$H_2 + F_2 \longrightarrow 2H^+ + 2F$$

And the ions combine to form hydrogen fluoride

$$2H^+ + 2F \longrightarrow 2HF$$

$$H_2 + F_2 \longrightarrow 2HF$$

In many redox reaction, a catalyst can be used to accelerate slow reaction where as in some reactions heating and a slow addition of the titrant may be required near the end point.

An oxidising agent is a substance in a redox reaction that oxidize another reactant and itself reduced by removing electrons from that reactant. Common oxidizing agents are O_2 (oxygen), O_3 (ozone), H_2O_2 (hydrogen peroxides) etc.

A reducing agent is that which reduce another reactant and itself oxidized by donating electrons to that reactant. Common reducing agents are $LiAlH_4$ (lithium aluminium hydride), $NaBH_4$ (sodium borohydride).

Redox Indicators

A **redox indicator** (also called an **oxidation-reduction indicator**) is an indicator that undergoes a definite color change at a specific electrode potential

There are two common types of redox indicators:

metal-organic complexes (e.g., phenanthroline)

true organic redox systems (e.g., methylene blue)

Some redox titration does not require an indicator due to intense color of the constituents. For instance, in permanganometry a slight faint persisting pink color signals at the end point of the titration because of the color of the excess oxidizing agent potassium permanganate.

Experiment 2.1

To Prepare and Standardize 0.1N Potassium Permanganate Solution

Theory

Standardization of potassium permanganate involves oxidation reduction reaction. Potassium permanganate is a strong oxidizing agent and oxalic acid is a reducing agent. The reaction between potassium permanganate and oxalic acid tends to proceed slowly, thus warming at 70 $^{\circ}$C is required. It is kept in tightly closed containers and must be handled with care because it may explode when brought in contact with readily oxidizable substances.

Chemical reaction

$$5\ H_2C_2O_4 \cdot 2H_2O + 2KMnO_4 + 2H_2SO_4 \longrightarrow K_2SO_4 + 2MnSO_4 + 18H_2O + 10CO_2$$

Oxalic acid   Potassium permanganate   Potassium sulphate   Manganese sulphate

Chemicals required

1. 0.1N potassium permanganate solution: Add 15.8 g $KMnO_4$ in 500 mL of distilled water. Boil the solution for one hour, cool and filter it and make the volume up to 1000 mL.

2. 0.1N Oxalic acid: Add 6.3 g of oxalic acid in 500 mL of distilled water in a 1000 mL volumetric flask. Dissolve and make up the volume of the solution up to 1000 mL mark with distilled water.

3. Sulphuric acid.

Procedure

1. Pipette out 20 mL of 0.1 N oxalic acid solution into a conical flask.
2. Add 5 mL of concentrated sulphuric acid slowly to the solution.
3. Warm the solution up to 70 $^{\circ}$C on water bath.
4. Fill the burette with given potassium permanganate solution.

5. Titrate the solution in conical flask with potassium permanganate by slowly adding the solution from the burette.

6. With first few drops pink color appears which persists for 20 sec.

7. Wait till the color disappears and then continue the titration.

8. The end point is obtained when a light pink color persists for about 30 sec even after shaking the flask.

Observation and Calculations

Normality of potassium permanganate

$$N_1V_1 = N_2V_2$$

where,

N_1 = normality of oxalic acid (0.1N), V_1 = volume of 0.1N oxalic acid (10 mL)

N_2 = normality of $KMnO_4$, V_2 = volume of $KMnO_4$ used (X ml)

$$N_2 = \frac{N_1V_1}{V_2} = \frac{0.1 \times 10}{X} = Y$$

Experiment 2.2

To Prepare and Standardize 0.1M Potassium Permanganate and Perform Assay of Hydrogen Peroxide

Theory

Hydrogen peroxide is a strong oxidizing agent and evolves nascent oxygen. Hydrogen peroxide and acidified potassium permanganate, both are oxidizing agents. They reduce each other and with the evolution of gaseous oxygen. Hydrogen peroxide being stronger oxidizing agent reduce potassium permanganate and causes its discoloration. At the end point, excess drops of potassium permanganate gives pink color to the solution acting as a self indicator.

Chemical reaction

$$2KMnO_4 + 3H_2SO_4 + 5H_2O_2 \longrightarrow K_2SO_4 + 8H_2O + SO_2 + 2MnSO_4$$

| Potassium permanganate | Hydrogen peroxide | Potassium sulphate | Manganese sulphate |

Chemicals required

1. **0.1M potassium permanganate solution:** Add 15.8 g $KMnO_4$ in 500 mL of distilled water. Boil the solution for one hour, cool and filter it and make the volume up to 1000 mL.

2. Sodium oxalate.

3. 1.0M Sulphuric acid solution. Add 30.0 mL of sulphuric acid in 900 mL of water. Make up the volume up to 1000 mL.

Procedure

1. **Standardization of 0.1M potassium permanganate solution:**

   (i) Weigh about 0.15 g of sodium oxalate and transfer it to 500 mL conical flask.

   (ii) Add 200 mL water and 50 mL 1.0M sulphuric acid solution to the conical flask.

   (iii) Boil the solution on hot plate.

   (iv) Now, titrate with potassium permanganate by adding the solution drop wise from burette.

   (v) Continue titration until pink color persists for 30 sec at the end point.

2. Assay of hydrogen peroxide

   (i) Pipette out 25.0 mL of hydrogen peroxide and transfer it to a 250 mL volumetric flask.

   (ii) Make up the volume of the solution up to 250 mL mark with distilled water and mix the solution thoroughly.

   (iii) Transfer 25.0 mL of diluted hydrogen peroxide into a conical flask.

   (iv) Add 10 mL of sulphuric acid solution.

   (v) Add standardized potassium permanganate solution to burette.

   (vi) Titrate the solution in conical flask with potassium permanganate solution

   (vii) Continue titration until the appearance of pink color at the end point.

   (viii) Take three concordant readings.

Observation and Calculations

1. Standardization of 0.1M potassium permanganate solution

Molarity of $KMnO_4$ solution = weight of sodium oxalate (g) × 0.4

     134 × volume of $KMnO_4$ solution (L)

The factor 0.4 is required because 5 moles of oxalate reacts with 2 moles of MnO_4^- (1 mole = 0.4 mole)

2. Assay of hydrogen peroxide

1 ml of 0.1M $KMnO_4$ solution = 0.001701 g of H_2O_2

Dilution factor = 10

V = mL of $KMnO_4$ solution used in titration

Amount of H_2O_2 (*w/v*) in 25 H_2O_2 (undiluted) =

$$\frac{V \times \text{Molarity (cal)} \times (0.001701) \times 10}{\text{Molarity (known)}}$$

% purity of H_2O_2 (*w/v*) =

$$\frac{V \times \text{Molarity (cal)} \times (0.001701) \times 10 \times 100}{\text{Molarity (known)} \times 25}$$

Experiment 2.3

To Determine Percentage Purity of Sodium Nitrite using Potassium Permanganate

Theory

Sodium nitrate ($NaNO_2$) solution cannot be placed in a flask because nitrous acid produced reacts slowly with $KMnO_4$ and can be lost therefore it is placed in the burette. If potassium permanganate ($KMnO_4$) solution turns brown or decomposes during titration, repeat the experiment.

Chemical equation

$$10\ NaNO_2 + 4\ KMnO_4 + 11\ H_2SO_4 \longrightarrow 10\ HNO_3 + 4\ MnSO_4 + 2K_2SO_4 + 5\ Na_2SO_4 + 6\ H_2O$$

Chemicals required

1. Sodium nitrite.
2. **0.1M $KMnO_4$:** Add 15.8 g $KMnO_4$ in 500 mL of distilled water. Boil the solution for one hour, cool and filter it and make the volume up to 1000 mL.
3. Concentrated sulphuric acid.

Procedure

1. Weigh about 0.6-0.7 g of the sample in a 250 mL graduated flask. Dissolve it in recently boiled and cooled water and make up the volume to get approximately 0.1M solution.
2. Place this solution in a burette.
3. Pipette 25 mL of 0.1M $KMnO_4$ into a conical flask and add 30 mL of water. Now add 4-5 mL of concentrated H_2SO_4 while rotating the flask and note the rise in temperature which should not be more than 40 °C.

4. Titrate this solution against sodium nitrate while maintaining the temperature of 40 °C.

5. The flask should be rotated during titration because HNO_2 reacts slowly with $KMnO_4$ at 40 °C or otherwise it will be lost as oxides of nitrogen.

6. The higher temperature will decompose $KMnO_4$.

7. When the color of the titrated solution becomes pale pink, raise the temperature and continue the addition of $NaNO_2$ drop-wise.

8. Towards the end of the titration the solution should be boiling.

Observation and Calculations

Weight of sample taken = W g

1 mL of 0.1M $KMnO_4$ solution = 0.003450 g of sodium nitrite

V = mL of $KMnO_4$ solution used in titration

$$\% \text{ purity of sodium nitrite} = \frac{V \times \text{Molarity (cal)} \times (0.003450)}{\text{Molarity (known)} \times W} \times 100$$

Experiment 2.4

To Prepare and Standardize 0.05N Ceric Ammonium Sulphate

Theory

Ceric Ammonium sulphate in the presence of dilute sulphuric acid is a powerful oxidizing agent. Unlike potassium permanganate which have several oxidation states, ceric salt have only one oxidation state. Ceric sulphate is a bright yellow colored salt and the cerous salt is colorless. As a practical oxidizing agent cerous sulphate has many advantage over permanganate and dichromate e.g.,

(i)   solutions are stable even on boiling and do not need protection from light,

(ii) reacts quantitatively with oxalate and arsenite, so that sodium oxalate and arsenic trioxide can be used as primary standard and

(iii) cerous ion is colorless and thus do not interfere with the indicator.

Chemical equation

$$Ce^{4+} + \bar{e} \ \rightleftharpoons \ Ce^{3+}$$

$$\underset{\text{ions}}{\text{Ceric}} \qquad\qquad \underset{\text{ions}}{\text{Cerium}}$$

Chemicals required

1. Ceric ammonium sulphate
2. Arsenic trioxide
3. 0.2M sodium hydroxide
4. Sulphuric acid
5. Osmium tetraoxide
6. Ferroin sulphate

Procedure

(i) Weigh accurately about 0.2 g of arsenic trioxide and transfer it to a conical flask.

(ii) Dissolve it by gentle heating in 15 mL of 0.2M sodium hydroxide.

(iii) Add 50 mL of 0.2M sulphuric acid solution, 0.15 mL of 2.5 mg/mL solution of osmium tetraoxide in sulphuric acid and 0.1 mL of ferroin sulphate.

(iv) Add the given ceric ammonium sulphate solution to the burette.

(v) Titrate the mixture with ceric ammonium sulphate by adding the solution drop wise from burette.

(vi) Continue the titration until red color disappears at end point.

Observation and Calculations

Molecular weight of arsenic trioxide = 197.84 g

Weight of arsenic trioxide = 0.1984 g

Volume of ceric ammonium sulphate solution consumed = 30.00 ml

M moles of arsenic trioxide = weight of arsenic trioxide (mg)/mol. weight of arsenic trioxide

From the above equation:

4 moles of Ce^{4+} = 1 mole of sodium arsenate

So, 1 mole of sodium arsenate = 4 Ce^{4+}

1.002 moles of sodium arsenate = 4 × 1.002 = 4.008 m moles of Ce^{4+}

Molarity of Ce^{4+} = m moles of Ce^{4+}/ml ceric ammonium sulphate
$$= 4.008/30 = 0.133M$$

Experiment 2.5

To Perform Assay of Ferrous Sulphate using Ceric Ammonium Sulphate

Theory

Assay of ferrous sulphate involves oxidation-reduction titration. Ferrous sulphate being a reducing agent gets oxidized to ferric sulphate by reaction with ceric ammonium sulphate (oxidizing agent). At the end point, with excess drops of ceric ammonium sulphate, ferroin sulphate (red color) gets oxidized to its ferric form giving blue color to the solution.

Chemical equation

$$2FeSO_4 + 2Ce(SO_4)_2 \cdot 2(NH_4)_2\,SO_4 \longrightarrow Fe_2(SO_4)_3 + Ce_2(SO_4)_3 + 2MnSO_4 + 4(NH_4)_2SO_4$$

Ferrous sulphate   Ceric ammonium sulphate   Ferric sulphate

Ferroin (Red color)   Ferrin (Blue color)

Chemicals required

1. **0.1M Ceric ammonium sulphate solution:** Dissolve 63.26 g of ceric ammonium sulphate in a mixture of 500 mL water and 30 mL sulphuric acid. Cool the solution and dilute it up to 1000 mL with water.

2. Ferroin sulphate

3. Sulphuric acid

4. Arsenic trioxide

Procedure

1. **Standardization of 0.1M ceric ammonium sulphate:**
   (i)   Weigh accurately about 0.2 g of arsenic trioxide and transfer it to a conical flask.
   (ii) Dissolve it in 15 mL of 0.2M sodium hydroxide solution by gentle heating.
   (iii) Add this solution to a mixture of 50 mL of 10% sulphuric acid solution, 0.15 mL of 2.5 mg/mL of osmium trioxide in 10% sulphuric acid and 0.1 mL of ferroin sulphate indicator.
   (iv) Fill the burette with ceric ammonium sulphate solution up to mark.
   (v)   Titrate the mixture slowly with given ceric ammonium sulphate by slowly adding the solution from burette.
   (vi) Continue titration until the appearance of red color at the end point.

2. **Assay of ferrous sulphate**
   (i)   Weigh accurately 0.5 g of ferrous sulphate and transfer it to a conical flask.
   (ii) Dissolve it in a mixture of 25 mL dilute sulphuric acid and 25 mL distilled water.
   (iii) Add a few drops of ferroin sulphate indicator.
   (iv) Titrate the mixture with 0.1M ceric ammonium sulphate by adding the solution drop wise from the burette.
   (v)   Continue titration till the blue color persists for 30 sec at the end point.

Observation and Calculations

1. Standardization of 0.1M ceric ammonium sulphate:

Molecular weight of arsenic trioxide = 197.84 g

Weight of arsenic trioxide used = 0.1984 g

Volume of ceric ammonium sulphate solution consumed = 30.00 mL

M moles of arsenic trioxide = weight of arsenic trioxide (mg)/mol. weight of arsenic trioxide

From the above equation:

4 moles of Ce^{4+} = 1 mole of sodium arsenate

So, 1 mole of sodium arsenate = 4 Ce^{4+}

1.002 moles of sodium arsenate

$$= 4 \times 1.002 = 4.008 \text{ m moles of } Ce^{4+}$$

Molarity of Ce^{4+} = m moles of Ce^{4+}/ml ceric ammonium sulphate

$$= 4.008/30 = 0.133 \text{ M}$$

2. Assay of ferrous sulphate

% purity of ferrous sulphate =

$$\frac{0.0278 \times \text{vol. of cerric amm. sulphate used} \times \text{molarity (cal)}}{\text{Weight of ferrous sulphate taken} \times \text{molarity (known)}}$$

Experiment 2.6

To Perform Assay of Ferrous Fumarate using Ceric Ammonium Sulphate

Theory

Ferrous fumarate, is the iron (II) salt of fumaric acid, occurring as a reddish-orange powder and it is used to supplement iron intake. Its assay is done by redox titration by using ceric ammonium sulphate and solution of ferroin sulphate is used as indicator. In the presence of ferrous ions, the color of the indicator changes from orange red to pale green on formation of ferric ions.

Chemicals required

1. **0.1M Ceric ammonium sulphate solution:** Dissolve 63.26 g of ceric ammonium sulphate in a mixture of 500 mL water and 30 mL sulphuric acid. Cool the solution and dilute it up to 1000 mL with water.
2. Ferroin sulphate
3. Sulphuric acid
4. Arsenic trioxide
5. Ferrous fumarate

Procedure

1. **Standardization of 0.1M ceric ammonium sulphate**
   (i) Weigh accurately about 0.2 g of arsenic trioxide and transfer it to a conical flask.
   (ii) Dissolve it in 15 mL of 0.2M sodium hydroxide solution by gentle heating.
   (iii) Add this solution to a mixture of 50 mL of 10% sulphuric acid solution, 0.15 mL of 2.5 mg/mL of osmium trioxide in 10% sulphuric acid and 0.1 mL of ferroin sulphate indicator.

(iv) Fill the burette with ceric ammonium sulphate solution up to mark.

(v) Titrate the mixture slowly with given ceric ammonium sulphate by slowly adding the solution from burette.

(vi) Continue titration until the appearance of red color at the end point.

2. Assay of ferrous fumarate

(i) Weigh accurately 0.3 g of ferrous fumarate and transfer it to a conical flask.

(ii) Dissolve it in a mixture of 15 mL dilute sulphuric acid followed by heating.

(iii) Cool the mixture and add 50 mL of distilled water.

(iv) Add a few drops of ferroin sulphate indicator.

(v) Titrate the mixture with 0.1M ceric ammonium sulphate by adding the solution drop wise from the burette.

(vi) Continue titration till the blue color persists for 30 sec at the end point.

Observation and Calculations

1. Standardization of 0.1M ceric ammonium sulphate

Molecular weight of arsenic trioxide = 197.84 g

Weight of arsenic trioxide used = 0.1984 g

Volume of ceric ammonium sulphate solution consumed = 30.00 mL

M moles of arsenic trioxide = weight of arsenic trioxide (mg)/mol. weight of arsenic trioxide

From the above equation:

4 moles of Ce^{4+} = 1 mole of sodium arsenate

So, 1 mole of sodium arsenate = 4 Ce^{4+}

1.002 moles of sodium arsenate = 4 × 1.002 = 4.008 m moles of Ce^{4+}

Molarity of Ce^{4+}

$\qquad$ = m moles of Ce^{4+}/ml ceric ammonium sulphate

$\qquad$ = 4.008/30 = 0.133 M

2. Assay of ferrous sulphate

% purity of ferrous fumarate =

$$\frac{0.01699 \times \text{vol. of cerric amm.sulphate used} \times \text{molarity (cal)}}{\text{Weight of ferrous fumarate taken} \times \text{molarity (known)}}$$

Experiment 2.7

To Prepare and Standardize 0.1N Iodine Solution

Theory

In **iodimetry**, quantitative oxidation of reducing agents, such as arsenous acid (H_2AsO_3) may be carried out by employing standard solutions of iodine. This type of assay is known as **'direct method of iodimetry'**.

Chemical equation

$$As_2O_3 + 2H_2O \longrightarrow As_2O_5 + 4H^+ + 4e$$

$$As_2O_3 + 2I_2 + 2H_2O \rightleftharpoons As_2O_5 + 4H^+ + 4e$$

Chemicals required

1. Iodine solution
2. Hydrochloric acid
3. Arsenic trioxide
4. Starch mucilage indicator
5. Methyl orange indicator

Procedure

1. Weigh 0.2 g of arsenic trioxide and transfer it to a conical flask.
2. Dissolve it in 20 ml of 1.0N NaOH solution by gentle warming.
3. Add two drops of methyl orange.
4. Add sufficient quantity of dilute hydrochloric acid until yellow color changes to pink.
5. Now add 2 g of sodium bicarbonate to the conical flask.
6. Add 50 ml of water and starch mucilage as indicator.
7. Fill the burette with given iodine solution up to mark.
8. Titrate the mixture with given iodine solution until permanent blue color is produced.

Observation and Calculations

Normality of iodine

$$N = \frac{\text{Weight of arsenic trioxide}}{\text{ml of iodine consumed} \times 0.04946}$$

0.04946 is the milliequivalent weight of arsenic trioxide

Experiment 2.8

To Prepare and Standardize 0.1N Sodium Thiosulphate and Perform Assay of Copper Sulphate

Theory

This is an iodometry titration. It depends upon the instability of cupric iodide which is formed in first reaction. Due to instability, it get decomposed to give cuprous iodide with libration of free iodine in second reaction. The free iodine is titrated with 0.1N sodium thiosulphate. Starch indicator is added towards the end of titration as it forms stable complex with excess of iodine. Decomposition of cupric iodide to liberate cuprous iodide and iodine is a reversible reaction. To prevent this, potassium thiocyanate is added which reacts with cuprous iodide to form cuprous thiocyanate.

Chemical equation

$$2\ CuI_2 \longrightarrow Cu_2I_2 + I_2$$

$$I_2 + 2\ Na_2S_2O_3 \longrightarrow Na_2S_4O_6 + 2\ NaI$$

Sodium
thiosulphate

Chemicals required

1. Copper sulphate
2. Potassium iodide
3. 0.1 N Potassium iodate solution (prepared by dissolving 2.14 g of potassium iodate in 100 mL in distilled water)
4. Sodium thiosulphate (prepared by dissolving 2.48 g $Na_2S_2O_3$ and 0.2 g of sodium carbonate in 100 mL in distilled water)
5. Starch indicator

Procedure

1. Standardization of $Na_2S_2O_3$ solution

(i) Pipette out 10 mL of 0.1N potassium iodate in a clean iodine flask.

(ii) Add 2 g of potassium iodide and 5 mL of dil. H_2SO_4.

(iii) Keep the flask in dark for 10 min.

(iv) Fill the burette with 0.1N sodium thiosulphate solution up to mark.

(v) Titrate the content of the flask against 0.1N sodium thiosulphate solution by slowly adding the solution from burette using starch as an indicator.

(vi) Repeat the titration to get three concordant readings

(vii) Calculate the normality of sodium thiosulphate used.

2. Assay of copper sulphate

(i) Weigh accurately about 1.0 gm of sample and transfer it to a conical flask.

(ii) Dissolve in 50 mL of water.

(iii) Add 3 g of KI and 5 ml of acetic acid.

(iv) Fill the burette with 0.1N $Na_2S_2O_3$ solution up to mark.

(v) Titrate the librated iodine with 0.1N $Na_2S_2O_3$, using starch as indicator.

(vi) Continue titration until faint blue color remains.

(vii) Now add 2 g of potassium thiocyanate, stir well and continue the titration until the blue color disappears.

(viii) Report the titration for three readings. Calculate the % purity by using factor.

Observation and Calculations

1. Normality of sodium thiosulphate

$$N_1V_1 = N_2V_2$$

Where,

N_1 = normality of KIO_3 (0.1N), V_1 = volume of 0.1N KIO_3 (10 mL)

N_2 = normality of $Na_2S_2O_3$ (?), V_2 = volume of $Na_2S_2O_3$ used (X mL)

$$N_2 = \frac{N_1 V_1}{V_2} = \frac{0.1 \times 10}{X} = Y$$

2. Assay of copper sulphate

Equivalent Factor for each mL of 0.1N $Na_2S_2O_3$ = 0.02497g of $CuSO_4$.

$$\text{Percentage purity of } CuSO_4 = \frac{X \times 0.02497 \times 100 \times 0.1}{1.0 \times Y} = Z\%$$

Experiment 2.9

Determination of Ascorbic Acid using Potassium Iodate

Theory

Ascorbic acid gets oxidized by iodine in acidic medium. Assay of ascorbic acid using potassium iodate is a kind of back titration. Ascorbic acid can be determined by direct titration with acidified iodine solution. But low solubility of iodine makes this method unsuitable. In the present method, this drawback is resolved by reacting excess iodide with iodate which generates excess of iodine. The excess of iodine is back titrated with sodium thiosulphate solution.

Chemical equation

Ascorbic acid $+ I_2 \longrightarrow$ Dehydroascorbic acid $+ 2H^+ + 2I^-$

$$IO_3^- + 3I^- + 6H^+ \longrightarrow 3I_2 + 3H_2O$$

$$I_2 + 2S_2O_3^{2-} \longrightarrow 2I^- + S_4O_6^{2-}$$

Chemicals required

1. Ascorbic acid

2. **Standard 0.01M potassium iodate solution:** Weigh accurately 2.1 g potassium iodate and transfer it to a 1000.0 mL volumetric flask. Add 200 mL of distilled water and dissolve potassium iodate. Make up the volume of solution up to 1000 mL with distilled water.

3. **Standard 0.06M sodium thiosulphate:** Dissolve 0.05 g of sodium carbonate and 7.5 g of sodium thiosulphate pentahydrate in water and dilute it up to 500 mL in a volumetric flask.

4. Potassium iodide

5. 0.5M sulphuric acid solution. Add 30 mL of concentrated sulphuric acid to 970 mL of water

6. Starch indicator

Procedure

1. **Standardization of sodium thiosulphate**

   (i)   Weigh accurately about 1.3 g of potassium iodate and transfer to a 250 mL volumetric flask. Dissolve it in water and make up the volume up to 250 mL.

   (ii) Pipette out 25.0 mL of potassium iodate solution into a conical flask.

   (iii) Add 2 g of potassium iodide and 10 mL of 0.5M sulphuric acid.

   (iv) Titrate the solution immediately with sodium thiosulphate solution until the solution becomes pale yellow.

   (v)   Add 2 mL of starch solution and titrate until blue color appears at the end point.

2. **Assay of ascorbic acid**

   (i)   Dissolve 1 g of ascorbic acid in about 150 mL of 0.5M sulphuric acid.

   (ii) Transfer this solution to 250 mL volumetric flask and make up the volume up to 250 mL with distilled water.

   (iii) Pipette out 25.0 mL of ascorbic acid solution and transfer to a conical flask and add 5 mL of 1M potassium iodide solution.

   (iv) Pipette out 25.0 mL of standard potassium iodate solution and add to the above mixture.

   (v)   Excess iodine is immediately back titrated with standard sodium thiosulphate solution.

   (vi) Add a few drops of starch indicator when the reaction mixture turns pale yellow.

   (vii) Continue titration until blue color appears at end point.

Observation and Calculations

1. Total moles of iodine generated

$$IO_3^- \text{(aq.)} + 5I^- \text{(aq.)} + 6H^+ \text{(aq.)} \longrightarrow 3I_2 \text{(aq.)} + 3H_2O \text{(l)}$$

No. of moles of iodine $= 3 \times$ no. of moles of iodate ions **(A)**

2. Excess of unreacted iodine mole

$$I_2 \text{(aq.)} + \text{ascorbic acid} \longrightarrow \text{dehydroascorbic acid} +$$
$$2H + \text{(aq.)} + 2I^- \text{(aq.)}$$

No. of moles of iodine reacted with ascorbic acid $=$ **B**

$$I_2 \text{(aq.)} + \text{ascorbic acid} \longrightarrow \text{dehydroascorbic acid} +$$
$$2H + \text{(aq.)} + 2I^- \text{(aq.)}$$

No. of moles of thiosulphate $=$ **C**

No. of moles of excess iodine $=$ **D**

3. Calculation of reacted iodine moles

No. of moles of iodine reacted with ascorbic acid **(B)** $= 3A - \frac{1}{2}C$

4. Assay of ascorbic acid

Amount of ascorbic acid

$= $ No. of moles of ascorbic acid $\times\, 176 \times 10\ (250/25)$

Experiment 2.10

To Prepare and Standardize 0.1N Potassium Dichromate

Theory

Potassium dischromate ($K_2Cr_2O_7$) is a strong oxidizing agent, quite comparable to $KMnO_4$ that normally shows only one pertinent reduced oxidation state. Potassium dichromate exhibits much greater stability in aqueous solution in comparison to potassium permanganate. Potassium dichromate possesses an inherent orange color that is not intense enough to serve its own end-point signal, specifically in the presence of the green Cr^{3+} ion, which is supposed to be present at the end-point.

Chemical equation

$$K_2Cr_2O_7 + 4H_2SO_4 \longrightarrow K_2SO_4 + Cr_2(SO_4)_3 + 4H_2O + 3(O)$$

Potassium   Potassium   Chromium
dichromate   sulphate   sulphate

Chemicals required

1. 0.05N Mohr's salt
2. Sulphuric acid
3. 0.1N Potassium dichromate solution

Procedure

1. **Preparation of standard solution of Mohr's salt $FeSO_4$ $(NH_4)_2.SO_4. 6H_2O$**

   (i) Weigh accurately about 4.9 g of pure sample of Mohr's salt and transfer it to a 250 mL volumetric flask.

   (ii) Add 20 mL of dilute sulphuric acid (9N) and make up the volume to the mark with distilled water.

   (iii) Now mix the contents of the flask thoroughly.

2. Standardization of 0.1N $K_2Cr_2O_7$ Solution

(i)   Transfer 20 mL of the primary standard solution (Mohr's salt) to the titration flask.

(ii) Add 20 mL of 2N sulphuric acid.

(iii) Take the potassium dichromate solution in the burette.

(iv) Soak and dry a filter paper with freshly prepared K_3 [Fe $(CN)_6$] solution.

(v)   Now, proceed with the titration of Mohr's salt solution against $K_2Cr_2O_7$ solution.

(vi) Transfer drops of the titrated solution by means of a glass rod on the filter paper soaked with indicator.

(vii) End point is reached when green color appears on applying few drops of the titrated solution by means of a glass rod on the filter paper soaked with indicator.

Observation and Calculations

1. Preparation of standard solution of Mohr's salt $FeSO_4(NH_4)_2.SO_4.6H_2O$

The quantity of Mohr's salt required for 250 mL of the solution with a normality of 0.05N can be calculated as follows:

$$\text{Mohr's salt} = \frac{\text{Eq. wt. of Mohr's salt} \times \text{volume} \times 0.05}{1000}$$

or $= 4.9$ g

2. Standardization of 0.1N $K_2Cr_2O_7$ Solution

Normality of potassium dichromate can be calculated using the relationship:

$$N_1V_1 \ (K_2Cr_2O_7) = N_2V_2 \ (\text{Mohr's salt})$$

CHAPTER 3

Precipitation Titration

Precipitation Titration

The precipitation titrations are those type of titration in which the titrant forms a precipitate with the analyte. These titrations are also termed as argentimetric processes. The basis of these titrations could be made by numerous precipitation reactions. The basic requirements of these precipitation reactions are; It must be sufficiently rapid and complete, lead to a product of reproducible composition and of low solubility. Some difficulties found in these titrations are:

1. Precipitation frequently proceeds slowly or starts after some time.

2. Sometimes precipitate adsorb and thereby co-precipitate the species being titrated or the titrant.

3. The indicator used may also be adsorbed on the precipitate formed during the titration and thereby unable to function properly at the end point.

4. If dark color precipitates are formed, then visual detection of color change at the end point is near to the impossible and even if white precipitate is formed, the milky solution may still make visualization of end point difficult.

Due to all these problems, these precipitation titrations are not so popular in present days for analysis.

Volhard's Method

This method was first described by the **"Jacob Volhard"**, a German Chemist, in 1874. This is an indirect titration procedure used for determining the anions that precipitate with silver. When a standard solution of ammonium or potassium thiocyanate is added from a burette to a solution of silver salt in the presence of nitric acid and ferric alum indicator in the titration flask, a precipitate of silver thiocyanate continues to be formed until the silver gets completely precipitated.

$$Ag^+ + CNS^- \longrightarrow Fe(CNS)_3$$
$$Red$$

The addition of a further drop of thiocyanate reacts with the ferric ion to form a red colored ferric thiocyanate complex

$$Fe^{3+} + 3\,CNS^- \longrightarrow Fe\,(CNS)_3$$
$$Red$$

The end point is the appearance of reddish brown coloration.

Conditions for Volhard's Method

1. The titration must perform in acidic medium to prevent the precipitation of iron (III) as hydrated oxide.

2. The indicator concentration should not be more than 0.2M.

3. In case of I^-, indicator should not add until all I^- is precipitated with Ag^+, since it would be oxidized by the Fe (III).

$$2\,Fe^{3+} + 2I \longrightarrow 2\,Fe^{2+} + I_2$$

4. If the silver halide ppt. is less soluble than AgSCN, they do not need to remove before titrating with SCN. Such is the case with I^-, Br^-.

5. If the silver halide ppt. are more soluble, it will react with the titrant which result in the over consumption of SCN and cause the diffuse end point. Such is the case with Cl^-

$$AgCl + SCN \longrightarrow AgSCN + Cl$$

To prevent this error (a) the precipitate must be filtered off before titrating with SCN; (b) add some volume of organic liquid like chloroform, nitrobenzene etc. which form a film around the precipitate; (c) use tartrazine as an indicator.

Applications

Volhard method can be used for determination of:

- Halides (I-, Cl-, Br-)
- Anions like phosphate, chromate, sulphide etc.
- Potassium as potassium tetraphenyl borate
- Fluoride as lead chloro fluoride

Advantages

- This method is useful where titrations have to be performed at low pH.

- The strong acidic environment give advantage for halide analysis because ions like carbonate, oxalate and arsenate do not interfere.

- Give accurate results due to back titrations.

Limitations

- This method cannot be used where the solutions has to be neutral.

- Time consuming

- Sometimes adsorption of Ag^+ may give false end point

Mohr's Method

This method was developed by Mohr in 1856 using potassium chromate as an indicator. This method involves the titration of silver nitrate against halides in neutral solution using 2% solution of potassium chromate as an indicator. The end point is marked by appearance of brick red precipitates due to the formation of silver chromate with excess of silver nitrate.

This method is based on the fact that silver halide is more soluble than silver chromate. Hence as long as there is any chloride or bromide left in the solution, no silver chromate is formed. Infact, even if formed, will immediately change to silver chloride or bromide by interaction with chloride or bromide e.g.,

$$Ag_2CrO_4 + 2Cl \longrightarrow 2\,AgCl + CrO_4^{2}$$

When whole of the chloride has been used up, silver chromate will be formed and brick red coloration or precipitate will appear.

Limitations

1. Silver chromate is soluble in acid, therefore the solution to be titrated, should be neutral. If acidic, it is first neutralized by adding pure powdered calcium carbonate and then indicator is added.

2. If the solution is alkaline, then silver nitrate is precipitated as silver hydroxide. In such cases, alkali is first neutralized by dilute nitric acid. The excess of the acid is then destroyed by adding pure powdered calcium carbonate.

3. Mohr's method is not suitable for iodides because of some adsorption difficulties and also difficulty in detecting the end point

as silver iodide precipitate is yellow colored like potassium chromate solution.

Fajan's Method

The end point in many precipitation titrations can be detected through the use of an adsorption indicator. Adsorption indicator methods were first developed by Fajans. Dichlorofluorescein, a weak organic acid, may be used for the titration of chloride with silver(I). The dichloro-fluoresceinate anion tends to be adsorbed on the surface of precipitated silver chloride, but not so strongly as chloride. In the first stages of a titration, chloride ions in solution are adsorbed preferentially on the surface of the precipitate.

As the titration proceeds, the chloride ion concentration decreases until it approaches a small value at the equivalence point. After the equivalence point a slight excess of the silver ion is present, and the attraction between adsorbed silver ion and dichlorofluoresceinate anion causes the latter to be adsorbed onto the surface of the precipitate. This adsorbed layer is pink, and the appearance of this pink color on the precipitate is taken to be the end point. Because the color change takes place on the surface of the precipitate, it is sharper if the surface area is large. Certain compounds, such as dextrin, keep precipitates of silver halides from coagulating and provide the needed surface area.

Experiment 3.1

To Prepare and Standardize Silver Nitrate

Theory

This method involves the titration of silver nitrate against halides in neutral solution using potassium dichromate as an indicator. The end point is marked by the appearance of a brick red precipitate or coloration due to the formation of silver chromate with an excess of silver nitrate.

Chemical equation

$$2Ag^+ + CrO_4^{2-} \longrightarrow Ag_2CrO_4 \downarrow$$

Silver chromate
(brick red ppt)

Reagents required

1. Sodium chloride
2. Silver nitrate solution
3. Potassium dichromate solution

Procedure

1. **Standardization of silver nitrate solution**

    (i) Pipette out 10 mL of 0.1M NaCl solution (prepared by dissolving 2.922 g in 500 mL of distilled water) in a clean flask.

    (ii) Add 1mL of potassium chromate indicator.

    (iii) Titrate the content of the flask against 0.1M $AgNO_3$ solution (prepared by dissolving 1.7 g of silver nitrate in 100 mL in distilled water) until brick red colored precipitate is formed.

    (iv) Repeat the titration to get three concordant readings

    (v) Calculate the normality of $AgNO_3$ used.

Observation and Calculations

$$\text{Molarity of AgNO}_3 = \frac{W}{58.44 \times V(\text{in liter})}$$

where, W = weight of sodium chloride in g

V = volume of silver nitrate solution consumed in liter

58.44 = molecular weight of sodium chloride

Experiment 3.2

To Prepare and Standardize Ammonium Thiocyanate by Volhard's Method

Theory

It is precipitation titration in which primary standard silver nitrate is used to standardize 0.1N ammonium thiocyanate solution, using ferric alum indicator. When a standard solution of ammonium thiocyanate is added from a burette to a solution of silver nitrate in the presence of nitric acid and ferric alum indicator in the titration flask, a precipitate of silver thiocyanate continues to be formed until the silver gets completely precipitated.

Chemical equation

$$SCN^- + Ag \longrightarrow AgSCN$$

Reagents required

1. Ammonium thiocyanate
2. Silver nitrate
3. Nitric acid
4. Ferric ammonium sulphate solution

Procedure

1. Pipette out 10 mL of 0.1M silver nitrate solution in a clean conical flask.

2. Dilute with 50 mL of water and add 2 mL of nitric acid and 2 mL of ferric ammonium sulphate solution.

3. Titrate the content of the flask against 0.1M ammonium thiocyanate solution (prepared by dissolving 0.76 g ammonium thiocyanate in 100 mL in distilled water) until the red brown color is appear.

4. Repeat the titration to get three concordant readings

5. Calculate the normality of ammonium thiocyanate used.

Observation and Calculations

The molarity of is calculated by:

$$M_1V_1 = M_2V_2$$

where,

M_1 = molarity of silver nitrate (0.1M), V_1= volume of 0.1M silver nitrate (10 mL)

$$M_2 = \frac{M_1V_1}{V_2} = \frac{0.1 \times 10}{X} = Y$$

M_2 = molarity of NH_4SCN (?), V_2 = volume of NH_4SCN used (X mL)

Experiment 3.3

To Determine Sodium Chloride by Mohr's Method

Theory

Sodium chloride is an example of electrolyte replenisher. It is assayed by Mohr's method. In this method, the sample is dissolved in water and titrated against a standard solution of $AgNO_3$ using potassium chromate as indicator. At the end-point it gives brick red colored precipitates are due to the formation of silver chromate.

Chemical equation

$$NaCl + AgNO_3 \longrightarrow NaNO_3 + AgCl$$

Sodium chloride   Silver nitrate   Sodium nitrate   Silver chloride

$$AgNO_3 + K_2Cr_2O_7 \longrightarrow KNO_3 + Ag_2CrO_4$$

Potassium dichromate   Silver chromate

Reagents required

1. Sodium chloride

2. Silver nitrate solution

3. Potassium dichromate solution

Procedure

1. Standardization of silver nitrate solution

    (i) Pipette out 10 mL of 0.1M NaCl solution (prepared by dissolving 2.922 g in 500 mL of distilled water) in a clean flask.

    (ii) Add 1 mL of potassium chromate indicator.

(iii) Titrate the content of the flask against 0.1M AgNO$_3$ solution (prepared by dissolving 1.7 g of silver nitrate in 100 mL in distilled water) until brick red colored precipitates are formed.

(iv) Repeated the titration to get three concordant readings

(v) Calculate the normality of AgNO$_3$ used.

2. For assay of sodium chloride

(i) Weigh accurately about 0.25 g of sample; dissolve in 50 mL of water.

(ii) Titrate the solution with 0.1N AgNO$_3$ solution using potassium chromate as indicator.

(iii) Report the titration for three readings. Calculate the % purity by using factor.

Observation and Calculations

1. Standardization of silver nitrate solution

$$\text{Molarity} = \frac{W(g)}{58.44 \times V(\text{in liter})}$$

where,   W = weight of sodium chloride (g)

V = volume of silver nitrate solution consumed in liter

58.44 = molecular weight of sodium chloride

2. For assay of sodium chloride

% of sodium chloride =

$$\frac{0.005844 \times \text{Vol. of silver nitrate used} \times \text{molarity (cal)} \times 100}{\text{Weight of the sample (g)} \times 0.1(\text{molarity given})}$$

Experiment 3.4

To Determine Chloride Ions by Fajan's Method

Theory

When an analyte Cl^- in a sample solution is titrated with Ag^+; the titration reaction would be

$$Ag^+ + Cl^- \longrightarrow AgCl$$

Silver chloride forms colloidal particles. Before the equivalence point, the surface of the precipitant particles will be negatively charged due to the adsorption of excess Cl^- to the surface of the particles. A diffuse positive counter-ion layer will surround the particles. When the equivalence point is reached, there is no longer an excess of analyte Cl^-, and the surface of the colloidal particles are largely neutral. After the equivalence point, there will be an excess of titrant Ag^+, some of these will adsorb to the solid AgCl particles, which will now be surrounded by a diffuse negative counter-ion layer. Adsorption indicators are dyes, such as dichlorofluorescein, that usually exist as anions in the titration solution. The doubly charged dichlorofluorescein anion is attracted into the counter-ion layer immediately following the equivalence point, when the surface charge of the particles changes from negative to positive.

Chemical equation

$$K_2Cr_2O_7 + 4H_2SO_4 \longrightarrow K_2SO_4 + Cr_2(SO_4)_3 + 4H_2O + 3(O)$$

Potassium dichromate   Potassium sulphate   Chromium sulphate

Chemicals required

1. 0.1M silver nitrate solution. Weigh about 8.5 g of silver nitrate in 500 mL of distilled water. Mix well and store in a dark bottle.

2. Sodium chloride

3. Dichlorofluorescein indicator. Dissolve 0.2 g of dichloro-fluorescein in 75 mL of ethanol and 25 mL of water.

Procedure

1. **Standardization of silver nitrate**

   (i)   Weigh about 1 g of sodium chloride from the container in the oven and transfer it to a glass bottle. Allow it to cool in dessicator for 15 min.

   (ii) Dry the unknown substance in an oven at 100 °C for 1 hr and then allow the unknown substance to cool to room temperature in dessicator. Weigh accurately 0.15-0.2 g of sodium chloride and dissolve it in 60 mL of distilled water.

   (iii) Add few drops of dichlorofluorescein indicator and 0.1 g of dextrin to the sodium chloride solution.

   (iv) Fill the burette with silver nitrate and immediately titrate sodium chloride solution with silver nitrate until first permanent pink color appears at the end point.

   (v)   Calculate the average molarity of silver nitrate.

2. **Titration of unknown substance**

   (i)   Weigh 0.2-0.3 g of the unknown sample.

   (ii) Titrate it similar to the standardization of silver nitrate solution.

   (iii) Repeat the titration to get three concordant readings.

Observation and Calculations

1. **Molarity of silver nitrate solution**

   Molarity =

   $$\frac{\text{Mass of sodium chloride (g)}}{\text{Mol. weight of sodium chloride} \times \text{volume of silver nitrate consumed (liter)}}$$

2. **% chloride in unknown sample**

   Moles Cl^- = Moles of silver nitare $\times$ volume of silver nitrate solution used

   Mass Cl^- = moles of Cl^- $\times$ atomic weight of Cl

   $$\% \text{ Cl} = \frac{\text{Moles of } Cl^- \times 100}{\text{Mass sample}}$$

CHAPTER 4

Gravimetric Analysis

Gravimetric analysis is a unique technique by means of which either an element or a compound is obtained in its purest form through isolation and subsequent weighing. In order to achieve this, the element or compound is first separated from a specific portion of the pharmaceutical substance being determined and consequently the weight of the constituent in the given sample is calculated on the basis of the weight of the product.

Gravimetric analysis is slow, tedious and time consuming in comparison to other volumetric analysis. However, this method gives good results. This method is applicable to only those substances which form metallic compounds on ignition and which do not contain volatile matter.

Gravimetric analysis involves the following steps:
   (i)   Precipitation
  (ii)   Filtration
 (iii)   Washing
  (iv)   Ignition
   (v)   Weighing

1. *Precipitation:* The anion or cation in a solution to be determined through gravimetric analysis is in a definite composition or leaves a residue of definite composition on ignition.

2. *Filtration:* Precipitates formed are separated from the solution by means of filtration either by filter paper, sintered crucible or gooch crucible. Different grades of filter papers are used for different precipitates. Ash-less filter paper is generally used.

3. *Washing:* Co-precipitated impurities, especially those on the surface, can be removed by washing the precipitate after filtering. An important consideration in this connection is the choice of washing liquid.

84

4. ***Drying or ignition:*** This process is to removes the solvent and wash electrolytes. If the collected precipitate is in a form suitable for weighing, it must be heated to remove the solvent and the absorbed electrolyte from the wash liquid. The preferable temperature use for drying is by drying it at 110°C to 120°C for 1 or 2 hours. Ignition at a higher temperature is required if a precipitate is converted to a more suitable form for weighing.

5. ***Weighing:*** The ignited precipitates are cooled and then placed in a dessicator so that they do not absorb moisture from atmosphere. Then they are weighed accurately on a chemical balance.

Applications of gravimetric method

Gravimetric methods have been developed for most inorganic anions and cations, as well as for such neutral species as water, sulfur dioxide, carbon dioxide and iodine. A variety of organic substances can also be easily determined gravimetrically. Examples include lactose in milk products, phenolphthalein in laxatives, nicotine in pesticides, cholesterol in cereals and benzaldehyde in almond extracts.

Limitations of gravimetric method

(i) Only a few derivatives are available which are quantitatively insoluble.

(ii) The impurities present in the sample are also converted to insoluble derivatives.

(iii) Washing of the precipitates to remove solvent and impurities, may dissolve some of the precipitates.

(iv) During filtration, some of the colloidal precipitates pass through the filter.

(v) Final drying of the precipitates to remove solvent, brings about the loss of precipitates by cracking.

Experiment 4.1

To Study Sintered Glass Crucible

Procedure

1. Sintered crucibles are made of resistance glass i.e., pyrex glass and have porous disc of sintered glass fused in the base of crucible.

2. These filter discs are of various porosities. These are of G_1, G_2, G_3, G_4 type. These pore sizes are 100-120, 40-50, 20-30 and 5-10 microns respectively.

3. Main feature of sintered glass crucibles are their resistance to chemicals and ease of dryness and cleaning.

4. These can be heated to 200°C.

5. If heated above 420°C, permanent strains are produced and they become soften above 160°C.

Observation and Calculations

Porosity	0	1	2	3	4	5
Pore diameter (μm)	200-250	100-120	40-50	20-30	5-10	1-2

Experiment 4.2

To Determine Water of Hydration in Crystalline Barium Chloride

Theory

Many ionic compounds which crystallize out of an aqueous solution have water molecules fixed in regular positions throughout the crystal lattice. These compounds are said to be hydrated and the number of water molecules per formula unit of the compound is shown as part of the formula. These water molecules of crystallization can be driven off by heating the hydrated compound. If the remaining compound has no water molecules of crystallization it is said to be anhydrous. The purpose of this experiment is to determine the number of water molecules of crystallization of hydrated barium chloride, $BaCl_2 \times H_2O$. A known mass of the hydrated compound will be heated so that the mass of water driven off can be determined.

Chemicals required

1. Barium chloride

Procedure

1. Weigh about 1.3933 g of anhydrous Barium chloride previously heated and dry it in china dish.

2. Place china dish with substance resting on low burner flame at height of 5-6 cm.

3. After few minutes, china dish may be heated by means of strong blue flame to dull redness.

4. Heating to dull redness at the end is done continuously for ten minutes.

5. Allow china dish to cool at room temperature and then transfer it to dessicator for 15 minutes and weigh the sample.

Observation and Calculations

Weight of empty china dish = X g

Weight of china dish + barium chloride = Y g

Weight of barium chloride = Y-X = Z g

After ignition,

Weight of barium chloride + china dish = A g

Weight of barium chloride = A – X = B g

Percentage of water of crystallization present in barium chloride

$$= (B/Z) \times 100 = Q \%$$

Experiment 4.3

To Determine Water of Crystallization in Copper Sulphate

Theory

Crystallization has long been one of the prime methods used to clean up impure compounds during reaction or synthetic sequences. It is a slightly crude process of salting out material by addition of an organic species and addition of simple selective reagent.

Reagents required

1. Copper sulphate

Procedure

1. Weigh small quantity of $CuSO_4$ and transfer to a china dish.
2. Heat the content on burner flame.
3. At the interval of few minutes, china dish may be heated by means of strong blue flame to dull redness.
4. Heating to dull redness at the end is done continuously for ten minutes.
5. Allow china dish to cool at room temperature and then transfer it to dessicator for 15 minutes and weigh.
6. Now weigh the sample.

Observation and Calculations

Weight of empty china dish = X g

Weight of china dish + $CuSO_4$ = Y g

Weight of $CuSO_4$ = Y – X = Z g

After ignition,

Weight of $CuSO_4$ + china dish = A g

Weight of $CuSO_4$ = A – X = B g

Percentage of water of crystallization present in $CuSO_4$

$$= (B/Z) \times 100 = Q\%$$

Experiment 4.4

To Determine Percentage of Chloride in Potassium Chloride

Theory

The experiment is based on the reaction that when silver nitrate solution is added to the chloride solution containing nitric acid, precipitates of silver chloride are formed which are then collected and dried to a constant weight.

Chemical equation

$$AgNO_3 + KCl \longrightarrow AgCl + KNO_3$$

| Silver nitrate | Potassium chloride | | Silver chloride | Potassium nitrate |

Chemicals required

1. Potassium chloride
2. Concentrated nitric acid
3. Silver nitrate

Procedure

1. Weigh accurately 0.2 g of potassium chloride and transfer it in a beaker.
2. Dissolve it in 150 mL of distilled water.
3. Add 0.5 mL of nitric acid and keep the solution in dark.
4. Now add 0.1N silver nitrate solution slowly with constant stirring.
5. Allow the precipitates to settle.
6. Heat the solution to boiling for 2-3 minutes until precipitates coagulate.
7. Cover the beaker and place it in dark for 1-2 hours.
8. Dry a clean sintered glass crucible to constant weight at 130-150°C.
9. Filter the solution through sintered glass crucible under suction.

10. Transfer all the precipitates to a crucible and wash with 0.1N nitric acid.
11. Finally wash the precipitates with water to remove all acid and then with small proportions of ethanol.
12. Heat the contents of the crucible at 130-150°C for 45 minutes, cool in dessicator and weigh.
13. Repeat heating and cooling until a constant weight is obtained.

CHAPTER 5

Non-aqueous Titration

Introduction

Non-aqueous is the titration of substances dissolved in non-aqueous solvents. It is the most common titrimetric procedure used in pharmacopoeial assays. The Bronsted Lowery theory of acid and bases can be applied equally well to reactions occurring during acid base titrations in non-aqueous solvents. Substances which give poor end points due to being weak acids or bases in aqueous solution will frequently give far more satisfactory end point when titrations are carried out in non-aqueous media. An additional advantage is that many substances, which are insoluble in water, are sufficiently soluble in organic solvents to permit their titrations in these non-aqueous media.

According to Bronsted Lowery theory, any acid, (HB) is considered to dissociate in solution to give a proton (H^+) and a conjugate base (B^-), whereas any base (B) will combine with a proton to produce a conjugate acid (HB^+):

$$HB \longleftrightarrow H^+ + B^-$$

$$B + H^+ \longleftrightarrow HB^+$$

The ability of substances to act as acids or bases will very much depend on the choice of solvent system. Non aqueous solvents are classified into the four groups: "aprotic, protophillic, photogenic and amphiprotic."

Merits of non aqueous over aqueous titrations: The substances, which are either to weakly acidic or too weakly basics to give sharp end point in aqueous solutions, can easily be titrated with accuracy is non-aqueous solvent.

Advantages of non aqueous solvent over aqueous solvent

1. Organic acids and bases that are insoluble in water, are soluble in non-aqueous solvent.

2. A non-aqueous solvent may help in titrating two or more acids in mixture. The individual acid can give separate end point in different solvent.

3. By the proper choice of the solvents or indicator, the biological ingredients of a substance whether acidic or basic can be selectively titrated.

4. Non aqueous titrations are simple and accurate.

Solvents used in non-aqueous titration

1. *Aprotic solvents:* Aprotic solvents include those substances, which may be considered chemically neutral and virtually un-reactive under the conditions employed. Carbon tetrachloride and toluene come in this group; they possess low dielectric constants, do not cause ionization in solutes and do not undergo reactions with acids and bases. Aprotic solvents are frequently used to dilute reaction mixture.

2. *Protophilic solvents:* Protophilic solvents are the substances that possess a high affinity for protons. The overall reaction can be represented as:-

$$HB + Sol. \rightleftharpoons Sol.H^+ + B^-$$

$$Acid + Basic\ solvent \rightleftharpoons Solvated\ proton + Conjugate\ base$$

The equilibrium in this reversible reaction will be generally influenced by the nature of the acid and the solvent. Weak acids are normally used in the presence of strongly protophilic solvents as their acidic strengths are then enhanced and then become comparable to these of strong acids; this is known as the **levelling effect.**

3. *Protogenic solvents:* Protogenic solvents are acidic in nature and readily donate protons. Anhydrous acids such as hydrogen fluoride and sulphuric acid fall in this category, because of their strength and ability to donate protons, they enhance the strength of weak bases.

4. *Amphiprotic solvents:* Amphiprotic solvents consist of liquids, such as water, alcohols and weak organic acids, which are slightly ionized and combine both protogenic and protophillic properties in being

able to donate protons and accept protons ethanoic acid (commonly called 'acetic acid') displays acidic properties in dissociating to produce protons:

$$CH_3COOH \longleftrightarrow CH_3COO^- + H^+$$

But in the presence of perchloric acid, a far stronger acid, it will accept a proton:

$$CH_3COOH + HClO_4 \longleftrightarrow CH_3COOH_2^+ + ClO_4^-$$

The $CH_3COOH_2^+$ ion can very readily give up its proton to react with a base, so basic properties of a base is enhanced and titrations between weak base and perchloric acid can often be accurately carried out using ethanoic acid as solvent.

5. *Levelling solvents:* In general, strongly protophilic solvents are important to force equilibrium equation to the right. This effect is so powerful that, in strongly protophillic solvents, all acids act as of similar strength. The converse occurs with strongly protogenic solvents, which cause all bases to act as they were of similar strength. Solvents, which act in this way, are known as **Leveling Solvents.**

Some Examples of Non-Aqueous Solvents

A very large number of organic solvents have been used for non-aqueous titrations, but a few have been used more frequently than others. Some of the most widely applied solvents systems are discussed below. In all instances pure, dry analytical reagent quality solvent should be used to assist in obtaining sharp end points.

1. *Glacial ethanoic acid:* Glacial ethanoic acid is the most frequently used non-aqueous solvent. Before it is used it is advisable to check the water content. This may be between 0.1% and 1.0%.

2. *Acetonitrile:* Acetonitrile (methyl cyanide, cyanomethane) is frequently used with other solvents such as chloroform and phenol and especially with ethanoic acid. It enables very sharp end points to be obtained in the titration of metal ethanoates when titrated with perchloric acid.

3. *Alcohol:* Salt of organic acids, especially of soaps are best determined in mixtures of glycols and alcohols or mixtures of glycols and hydrocarbons. The most common combinations are

ethylene glycol (dihydroxyethane) with propan-2-ol or butan-1-ol. The combinations provide admirable solvents for both the polar and non-polar ends of the molecules.

4. ***Dioxane:*** Dioxane is another popular solvent, which is often used in place of glacial ethanoic acid when mixtures of substances are to be quantified. Unlike ethanoic acid, dioxane is not a leveling solvent and separate end points are normally possible, corresponding to the individual components in the mixtures.

5. ***Dimethylformamide:*** Dimethylformamide (DMF) is a protophillic solvent, which is frequently employed for titrations between, for instance, benzoic acid and amides, although end points may sometimes be difficult to obtain.

Indicators for Non-aqueous Titrations

The ionized/unionized forms of indicators applies equally well for non-aqueous titrations but their color changes at the end point vary from titration to titrations, as they depend on the nature of the titrant. The color corresponding to the correct end point may be established by carrying out a potentiometric titration while simultaneously observing the color change of the indicator. The majority of non-aqueous titrations are carried out using a fairly limited range of indicators; here are some typical example.

1. ***Crystal violet:*** Used as 0.5% w/v solution in glacial acetic acid. Its color change is from violet through blue followed by green, then to greenish yellow, in reactions in which bases such as pyridine are titrated with perchloric acid.

2. ***Methyl red:*** Used as a 0.2% w/v solution in dioxane with a yellow to red color change.

3. ***Naphthol benzein:*** When employed as a 0.2% w/v solution in ethanoic acid gives a yellow to green color change. It gives sharp end points in nitro methane containing ethanoic anhydride for titration of weak bases against perchloric acid.

4. ***Quenaldine Red:*** Used as an indicator for drug determinations in dimethylformamide solution. A 0.1% w/v solution in ethanol gives a color change from purple red to pale green.

5. ***Thymol blue:*** Used extensively as an indicator for titrations of substances acting as acids in dimethyl formamide solution. A 0.2% w/v solution in methanol gives a sharp color change from yellow to blue at the end point.

Experiment 5.1

To Prepare and Standardize 0.1M Perchloric Acid

Theory

The acetic anhydride reacts with the water (approx. 30%) in perchloric acid and some traces in glacial acetic acid thereby making the resulting mixture practically anhydrous. Alkaline earth (*e.g.*, Mg, Ca, Ba) and alkali (*e.g.*, Na, K, Rb), salts of organic acids behave as bases in acetic acid solution.

$$RCOOM \rightleftharpoons RCOO^- + M^+$$

$$CH_2COOH_2 + RCOO^- \rightleftharpoons RCOOH + CH_3COOH$$

Onium ion   Acetic acid

In usual practice, potassium hydrogen phthalate (or potassium biphthalate, $KHC_8H_4O_4$) is employed as a standardizing agent for acetous perchloric acid.

Chemical reaction

Potassium hydrogen phthalate $+ HClO_4 \longrightarrow$ Phthalic acid $+ KClO_4$

Potassium hydrogen   Perchloric   Phthalic acid
phthalate   acid

Chemicals required

1. 8.5 mL of perchloric acid
2. 1 Liter of glacial acetic acid
3. 30 mL of acetic anhydride
4. Potassium hydrogen phthalate

Procedure

1. Preparation of perchloric acid

(i)   Gradually mix 8.5 mL of perchloric acid to 900 mL of glacial acetic acid with vigorous and continuous stirring.

(ii) Add 30 mL acetic anhydride and make up the volume to 1 liter with glacial acetic acid.

(iii) Allow the solution to stand for 24 hours before use.

2. Standardization of perchloric acid

(i)   Weigh accurately about 0.5 g of potassium hydrogen phthalate and transfer it to 100 mL conical flask.

(ii) Add 25 mL of glacial acetic acid into it.

(iii) Warm the solution until the salt gets completely dissolved.

(iv) Cool the solution.

(v)   Now add 2 drops of crystal violet indicator into conical flask.

(vi) Titrate the solution with 0.1M perchloric acid.

(vii) Continue the titration until solution turns bluish green at the end point.

Observation and Calculations

Standardization of perchloric acid

$$\text{Molarity of } HClO_4 \text{ solution} = \frac{\text{Weight of pot. hydrogen phthalate (g)}}{204 \times \text{volume of } HClO_4 \text{ used (mL)}}$$

where, 204 is the molecular weight of potassium hydrogen phthalate

Experiment 5.2

To Perform Assay of Metronidazole Benzoate Tablets I.P.

Theory

Metronidazole is a nitroimidazole antibiotic medication used particularly for anaerobic, bacteria and protozoa. It is chemically 2-(2-Methyl-5-nitroimidazol-1-yl) ethyl benzoate having empirical formula $C_{13}H_{13}N_3O_4$ and molecular weight 275.3 and is structurally

H$_3$C
N
N
NO$_2$
O
O

Metronidazole

Chemicals required

1. Metronidazole benzoate tablets
2. 0.1M perchloric acid
3. Glacial acetic acid
4. Potassium hydrogen phthalate
5. 0.1% brilliant green

Procedure

1. Preparation of perchloric acid

(i)   Gradually mix 8.5 mL of perchloric acid to 900 mL of glacial acetic acid with vigorous and continuous stirring.

(ii) Now add 30 mL acetic anhydride and make up the volume to 1 liter with glacial acetic acid.

(iii) Allow the solution to stand for 24 hours before use.

2. Standardization of perchloric acid

   (i) Weigh accurately about 0.5 g of potassium hydrogen phthalate and transfer it to 100 mL conical flask.

   (ii) Add 25 mL of glacial acetic acid into it.

   (iii) Warm the solution until the salt gets completely dissolved.

   (iv) Cool the solution.

   (v) Now add 2 drops of crystal violet indicator into conical flask.

   (vi) Titrate the solution with 0.1M perchloric acid.

   (vii) Continue the titration until solution turns bluish green at the end point.

3. Assay for Metronidazole benzoate tablets

   (i) Weigh and powder 20 Metronidazole Benzoate tablets and calculate their average weight.

   (ii) Weigh accurately about 0.25 g of Metronidazole Benzoate and transfer to a conical flask.

   (iii) Dissolve it in 50.0 mL of glacial acetic acid.

   (iv) Titrate with 0.1M perchloric acid using 0.1 % w/v brilliant green as indicator until yellowish green end point appears.

   (v) Perform a blank determination and make any necessary correction

Observation and Calculations

1. Standardization of perchloric acid

Molarity of $HClO_4$ solution

$$= \frac{\text{Weight of pot. hydrogen phthalate (g)}}{204 \times \text{volume of } HClO_4 \text{ used (mL)}}$$

where, 204 is the molecular weight of potassium hydrogen phthalate

2. Assay of Metronidazole benzoate

Weight of sample = W g

Volume of 0.1M perchloric acid used in Metronidazole titration = V_1 ml

Volume of 0.1M perchloric acid used in blank titration = V_2 mL

Difference $= V_1 - V_2 = V$ mL

Each ml of 0.1M perchloric acid $= 0.02753$ g of Metronidazole benzoate

$$\% \text{ of Metronidazole benzoate} = \frac{0.02753 \times V \text{ Molarity (cal)}}{\text{Molarity (given)} \times W} \times 100$$

Experiment 5.3

Determination of Percentage Purity of Diclofenac Sodium

Theory

Diclofenac sodium, 2-[2, 6-dichlorophenyl)-amino] benzene acetic acid monosodium salt, is a non-steroidal anti-inflammatory drug with potent activity and outstanding tolerability in the treatment of rheumatic disease. It is also used as an analgesic and antipyretic. This phenylacetic acid derivative acts as an inhibitor of diclofenac are those of potassium and diethyl-ammonium salt. Diclofenac is available as tablets (enteric coated, controlled release), creams and injectables. It is a weak base, hence titrated with acetous perchloric acid using crystal violet as indicator.

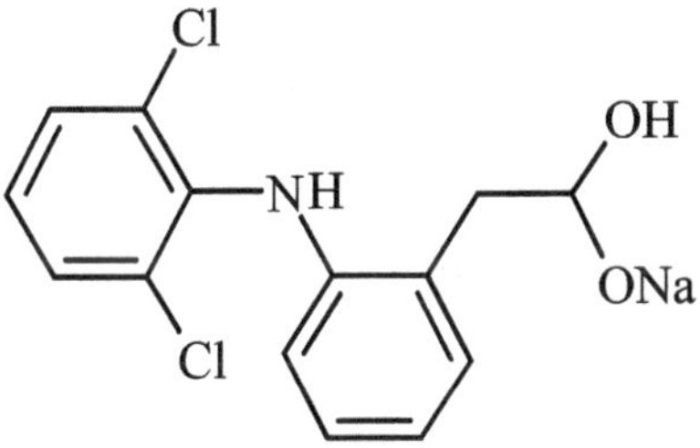

Diclofenac sodium

Chemicals required

1. 0.1M $HClO_4$ solution. To 900 mL of glacial acetic acid, add 8.5 mL of perchloric acid, mix, add 30 mL of acetic anhydride dilute to 1000 mL with glacial acetic acid, mix and allow to stand for 24 hours.
2. Potassium hydrogen phthalate.
3. Crystal violet indicator. Dissolve 0.2 g of crystal violet in 100 mL of acetic acid.
4. Glacial acetic acid.
5. Acetic anhydride.

Procedure

1. Standardization of 0.1M HClO$_4$ solution

(i) Weigh accurately about 350 mg of potassium hydrogen phthalate (KHP) and transfer it to conical flask.

(ii) Dissolve it in 50 mL of anhydrous acetic acid with gentle warming gently (if necessary).

(iii) Allow to cool and protect from air.

(iv) Titrate the above solution with the perchloric acid solution using 0.05 mL of crystal violet solution as indicator.

(v) Each mL of 0.1M perchloric acid = 20. 42 mg of C$_8$H$_5$KO$_4$.

Note: Restandardize perchloric acid before use. Store in amber bottle with well fitted suitable stoppers which prevent access to atmospheric carbon dioxide. Discard the solution after 30 days.

2. Determination of diclofenac sodium

(i) Weigh accurately about 0.2 g of diclofenac sodium and dissolve in 50 mL of glacial acetic acid.

(ii) Add few drops crystal violet indicator.

(iii) Titrate with 0.1M HClO$_4$ solution until green color.

(iv) Similarly, perform a blank titration.

Observation and Calculations

1. Standardization of perchloric acid

$$\text{Molarity of HClO}_4 = \frac{W(g)}{204 \times V(L)} \times 100$$

where   V = volume of perchloric acid consumed in mL.

           W = weight of potassium hydrogen phthalate in g.

           204 the molecular weight of KHP

2. Determination of diclofenac sodium

Molecular weight of diclofenac sodium = 318.14

Weight of sample = W g

The volume of 0.1M HClO$_4$ consumed in diclofenac sodium titration = V$_1$ mL

The volume of 0.1M HClO$_4$ consumed in blank titration = V$_2$ mL

Difference = $V_1 - V_2 = V$ mL

1 mole of diclofenac sodium = 1 mole of $HClO_4$ = 1000 mL of 1 mL $HClO_4$

Hence, each ml of 0.1M perchloric acid solution = 0.03181 g of $C_{14}H_{10}Cl_2NNaO_2$

The % of diclofenac sodium present in the sample is given by:

$$\% \text{ of Diclofenac sodium} = \frac{0.03181 \times V \times \text{Molarity(cal.)}}{\text{Molarity (given)} \times W} \times 100$$

Experiment 5.4

Determination of Percentage Purity of Methyldopa

Theory

Methyldopa is an antihypertensive drug. Methyldopa, the L-isomer of alpha-methyldopa, is levo-3-(3, 4-dihydroxyphenyl)-2-2methylalanine. Methyldopa is a white to yellowish white, odorless fine powder and is soluble in water.

Methyldopa

It is a weak base and so titrated with standard perchloric acid in glacial acetic acid.

Chemical equation

Methyldopa   Protonated methyldopa

Chemicals required

1. **0.1M perchloric acid:** To 900 mL of glacial acetic acid, add 8.5 mL of perchloric acid, mix, add 30 mL of acetic anhydride, dilute to 1000 mL with glacial acetic acid, mix and allow to stand for 24 hours.

2. Anhydrous formic acid.

3. Glacial acetic acid.

4. Dioxane.

5. Crystal violet indicator.

Procedure

1. Standardization of 0.1M perchloric acid solution

(i) Weigh accurately about 350 mg of potassium hydrogen phthalate (KHP) and transfer it to the conical flask.

(ii) Dissolve it in 50 mL of anhydrous acetic acid with gentle warming (if necessary).

(iii) Allow to cool protected from the air.

(iv) Titrate the above solution with the perchloric acid solution using 0.05 mL of crystal violet solution as indicator.

(v) Each mL of 0.1M perchloric acid =20.42 mg of $C_8H_5KO_4$.

2. Determination of methyldopa in tablet

(i) Weigh accurately about 0.2 g of sample and dissolve in a mixture of 15 mL of anhydrous formic acid, 30 mLof glacial acetic acid and 30 ml of dioxane.

(ii) Add 0.1 mL of crystal violet solution and titrate with 0.1M perchloric acid until the development of green color.

(iii) Perform a blank determination and make any necessary correction.

Observation and Calculations

1. Calculation of molarity of perchloric acid

$$\text{Molarity of } HClO_4 = \frac{W(g)}{204 \times V(L)}$$

where   V = volume of perchloric acid consumed in liter.

W = weight of potassium hydrogen phthalate in g.

204 the molecular weight of KHP.

2. Determination of methyldopa

Weight of sample = W g

The volume of 0.1M $HClO_4$ consumed = V mL

Each mL of 0.1 N perchloric acid solution = 0.02112 g of $C_{10}H_{13}NO_4$

The % of methyldopa present in the sample is given by:

$$\% \text{ of Methyldopa} = \frac{0.0211 \times V \times \text{Molarity (cal.)}}{\text{Molarity (given)} \times W} \times 100$$

Experiment 5.5

Determination of Percentage Purity of Ephedrine Hydrochloride

Theory

Ephedrine HCl is used as an expectorant bronchodilator. It is difficult to titrate halogen salt directly with acetic perchloric acid because there is no much difference in the proton attracting capabilities of the halide ion and perchlorate anions in glacial acetic acid. Therefore, the reaction does not proceed toward completion. Hence, mercuric acetate is added to ephedrine chloride to replace an equivalent amount of acetate ion which is readily protonated. Mercuric chloride remain un-dissociated in glacial acetic acid.

Chemical equation

$$2HClO_4 + 2CH_3COOH \longrightarrow 2CH_3COOH_2^+ + 2ClO_4^-$$

$$2C_{10}H_{15}N + HOCl + (Ac)_2 Hg \longrightarrow 2C_{10}H_{15}N + AcOH + HgCl_2$$

Ephedrine.HCl   Mercuric
                                 acetate

$$CH_3COO^- + CH_3COOH_2^+ \longrightarrow 2CH_3COOH$$

$$2C_{10}H_{15}N + AcOH + 2CH_3COOH_2^+ \longrightarrow 2C_{10}H_{10}N^+HO + 4CH_3COOH$$

Overall reaction

$$2C_{10}H_{15}N + HOCl^- + (Ac)_2Hg + 2HClO_4 \longrightarrow$$
$$2C_{10}H_{10}N^+H + AcOH + 2ClO_4^- + HgCl_2$$

Chemicals required

1. **0.1M solution of HClO$_4$ solution.** Dissolve 8.5 mL of 72 % HClO$_4$ in about 900 mL glacial acetic acid with constant stirring, add about 30 mL acetic anhydride and make up the volume (1000 mL) with glacial acetic acid and keep the mixture for 24 hour.

2. Crystal violet solution (0.2 % w/v in acetic acid).

3. Mercuric acetate solution (5 % w/v in acetic acid).

4. Glacial acetic acid

5. Acetic anhydride

6. Potassium hydrogen phthalate.

Procedure

1. **Standardization of the above prepared 0.1M HClO$_4$ solution**

    (i)   Weigh about 0.5 g of potassium acid phthalate (KHP) and transfer it to the conical flask.

    (ii) Add 25 mL of glacial acetic acid and add few drops of 5 % w/v crystal violet in glacial acetic acid as indicator.

    (iii) Titrate the solution with 0.1M HClO$_4$ solution till blue color appears.

    (iv) Each ml of 0.1N HClO$_4$ solution = 0.020414 g of potassium acid phthalate.

2. **Determination of ephedrine HCl content**

    (i)   Weigh accurately 20 tablets and find out the average weight of tablet.

    (ii) Grind the tablets to fine powder.

    (iii) Accurately weigh powder equivalent to about 0.15 gm of ephedrine hydrochloride and transfer it to the conical flask.

    (iv) Add glacial acetic acid (30 mL), mercuric acetate solution (10 mL) and crystal violet solution (0.1 mL) to it.

    (v)   Gently warm the solution, cool and titrate with 0.1M perchloric acid until the violet color changes to green blue.

    (vi) Perform a blank titration in the same way.

Observation and Calculation

1. **Standardization of the 0.1 M HClO$_4$ solution**

$$\text{Molarity of HClO}_4 = \frac{W(g)}{204 \times V(L)}$$

where V = volume of perchloric acid consumed in liter.

W = weight of potassium hydrogen phthalate in g.

204 is the molecular weight of KHP

2. **Determination of ephedrine HCl**

Weight of tablet powder = W g

The average weight of tablet = W_1 g

The volume of 0.1M HClO$_4$ solution consumed = V mL

From the equation:

1 mole of $C_{10}H_{15}NO.HCl = Cl^- + CH_3COO^- = HClO_4$

1000 mL of 0.1M HClO$_4$ solution = 201.7 g of ephedrine HCl

Each mL of 0.1M perchloric acid solution = 0.02017 gm of $C_{10}H_{15}NO.HCl$.

Experiment 5.6

Determination of Percentage Purity of Chlorpromazine

Theory

Chlorpromazine (10-[3-dimethylaminopropyl] phenothiazine) belongs to the primary chemical group of antipsychotic agents known as the phenothiazines. The determination of the chlorpromazine hydrochloride content is based on non-aqueous titration. Glacial acetic acid is used as the non-aqueous solvent and equivalence point is determined using visual indicators and potentiometer. The addition of mercuric acetate in the non-aqueous titrimetric method is based on the principle of removing the chloride counter ion so as to prevent the interface of the halide ion released by the titrant (acetous perchloric acid). The addition of mercuric acetate replaces the halide ion in chlorpromazine with a quantitative acetate ion which is a strong base in acetic acid. An intense red colored oxidation product is formed when ascorbic acid was not added. This made end-point detection with visual indicators to be difficult.

Chemicals required

1. 0.1M solution of $HClO_4$ solution. Dissolve 8.5 mL of 72% $HClO_4$ in about 900 mL glacial acetic acid with constant stirring, add about 30 mL acetic anhydride and make up the volume (1000 mL) with glacial acetic acid and keep the mixture for 24 hour.

2. Crystal violet solution (0.2 % w/v in acetic acid).

3. Mercuric acetate solution (5 % w/v in acetic acid).

4. Glacial acetic acid

5. Acetic anhydride

Procedure

1. Standardization of the above prepared 0.1M HClO₄ solution

   (i)   Weigh about 0.5 g of potassium acid phthalate (KHP) and transfer it to the conical flask.

  (ii)   Add 25 mL of glacial acetic acid and add few drops of 5 % w/v crystal violet in glacial acetic acid as indicator.

 (iii)   Titrate the solution with 0.1M HClO₄ solution till blue color appears.

 (iv)   Each ml of 0.1N HClO₄ solution = 0.020414 g of potassium acid phthalate.

2. Determination of chlorpromazine HCl in tablet

   (i)   Weigh accurately twenty tablets and reduce to fine powder.

  (ii)   From the powdered drug, take an amount equivalent to 0.35 g of chlorpromazine HCl and transfer into a 250 mL conical flask containing 50 mL of glacial acetic acid.

 (iii)   Shake the mixture and add 10 mL of 5 % w/v mercuric acetate, 2 g of ascorbic acid and 2 drops of 0.2 % w/v crystal violet indicator.

 (iv)   Stir the solution for 15 min with a magnetic stirrer and then titrate with 0.1M acetous perchloric acid to a blue end-point.

  (v)   Repeat the titration three times to get concordant reading.

Observation and Calculations

1. Standardization of the 0.1M HClO₄ solution

$$\text{Molarity of HClO}_4 = \frac{W(g)}{204 \times V(L)}$$

where   V = volume of perchloric acid consumed in liter.

         W = weight of potassium hydrogen phthalate in g.

2. Determination of Chlorpromazine HCl

Molecular weight of chlorpromazine HCl = 355. 78

Weight of tablet powder = W g

The average weight of tablet = W_1 g

The volume of 0.1 M $HClO_4$ solution consumed $= V$ mL

From the equation:

1 mole of $C_{17}H_{19}ClN_2S.HCl = Cl^- + CH_3COO^- = HClO_4$

1000 mL of 1.0M $HClO_4$ solution $= 355.3$ g of Chlorpromazine HCl

1 mL of 0.1M $HClO_4$ solution $= 0.03553$ g of chlorpromazine HCl

$$\% \text{ of Chlorpromazine} = \frac{0.03553 \times V \times \text{Molarity}\left(\text{cal.}\right)}{\text{Molarity}\left(\text{given}\right) \times W} \times 100$$

Experiment 5.7

To Prepare and Standardize 0.1M Sodium Methoxide Solution

Theory

Sodium methoxide is standardized by primary standard benzoic acid in dimethylformamide which enhances its acidity.

Chemical equation

$$C_6H_5COOH + HCON(CH_3)_2 \longrightarrow HCON^+H(CH_3)_2 + C_6H_5COO^-$$

$$CH_3ONa \longrightarrow CH_3O^- + Na^+$$

$$HCON^+H(CH_3)_2 + CH_3O^- \longrightarrow HCON(CH_3)_2 + CH_3OH$$

Overall reaction

$$C_6H_5COOH + CH_3ONa \longrightarrow C_6H_5COONa + CH_3OH$$

Benzoic acid   Sodium methoxide   Sodium benzoate   Methanol

Chemicals required

1. **0.1M Sodium methoxide solution:** Place 150 mL of MeOH in 100 mL volumetric flask and cool in ice. Add small portions (approximately 2.5 g) of freshly cut pieces of sodium metal. After addition of metal, add sufficient benzene to make 1000 mL and mix. Store in the reservoir of an automatic delivery burette protected from CO_2 and H_2O.

2. Dimethylformamide (DMF)

3. Azo-violet (0.1% *w/v* in DMF)

Procedure

1. Weigh accurately 400 mg of benzoic acid (primary standard) in a flask and dissolve in 80 mL of DMF.

2. Titrate the above solution with sodium methoxide using 3 drops of thymol blue (1% *w/v* DMF) as indicator

3. Continue the titration until the end point is blue.

4. Correct for the volume of $NaOCH_3$ solution consumed by 80 mL of DMF and calculate the molarity.

Observation and Calculations

$$\text{Molarity} = \frac{\text{Weight of Benzoic acid (g)}}{122 \times \text{Volume of sod. methoxide used (L)}} \times 100$$

where, 122 is the molecular weight of benzoic acid

Experiment 5.8

To Determine Percentage of Phenobarbitone

Theory

Phenobarbital (5-ethyl-5-phenylbarbituric acid or 5-ethyl-5-phenyl-hexahydro- pyrimindin-2,4,6-trione) is a barbiturate and the most widely used anticonvulsant worldwide

Chemical equation

$$O=C\begin{smallmatrix}NH-CO\\ \\NH-CO\end{smallmatrix}C\begin{smallmatrix}C_2H_5\\ \\C_2H_5\end{smallmatrix} + LiOMe$$

Phenobarbitone   Lithium methoxide

$$O=C\begin{smallmatrix}NH-CO\\ \\NH-CO\end{smallmatrix}C\begin{smallmatrix}C_2H_5\\ \\C_2H_5\end{smallmatrix} + CH_3OH$$

Chemicals required

1. Phenobarbitone
2. Dimethylformamide
3. Quinaldine red (0.1% w/v in ethanol)
4. Lithium methoxide

Procedure

1. Transfer 40 mL of DMF into a titration flask.
2. Add 3 drops of quinaldine red solution

3. Neutralize the above solution by titrating with N/10 lithium methoxide.

4. Accurately weigh 0.2 g of the drug sample in the flask.

5. Titrate with N/10 lithium methoxide using quinaldine red as indicator avoiding any contamination of lithium methoxide with H_2O and CO_2.

6. The end-point will be when the color changes from pink to colorless.

Observation and Calculations

0.02322 g of phenobarbitone $\equiv$ 1 mL of 0.1M lithium methoxide consumed

Experiment 5.9

To Determine the Percentage Purity of Ethosuximide

Theory

Ethosuximide is a weak acid so titrated with standard sodium methoxide solution in dimethylformamide which enhances acidity.

Chemical equation

Ethosuximide $+\ NaOCH_3\ \longrightarrow$ Sodium salt of ethosuximide $+\ CH_3OH$

Chemicals required

1. **0.1M sodium methoxide solution:** Place 150 mL of methanol in 1000 mL volumetric flask and cool it in ice water and add, in small portions, about 2.5 g of freshly cut sodium metal. The metal reservoir of an automatic delivery burette should be suitably protected from carbon dioxide and moisture.

2. Dimethylformamide.

3. Azo-violet (0.1 % w/v in DMF).

Procedure

1. **Standardization of above prepared 0.1M Sodium methoxide solution**

   (i) Weigh accurately 400 mg of benzoic acid (primary standard) in a flask and dissolve in 80 mL of DMF.

(ii) Titrate the above solution with sodium methoxide using 3 drops of thymol blue (1% *w/v* DMF) as indicator

(iii) Continue the titration until the end point i.e., appearance of blue color.

(iv) Correct for the volume of $NaOCH_3$ solution consumed by 80 mL of DMF and calculate the molarity.

2. Determination of ethosuximide

(i) Weight accurately about 0.2 g of the sample and dissolve in 50 mL of dimethylformamide.

(ii) Add 2 drops of Azo-violet solution and titrate with 0.1N sodium methoxide to a deep blue end point, taking precautions to prevent absorption of atmospheric carbon dioxide.

(iii) Perform a blank titration and make any necessary correction.

(iv) Each mL of 0.1N sodium methoxide is equivalent to 0.01412 g of $C_7H_{11}NO_2$.

Observation and Calculations

1. Determination of molarity of sodium methoxide solution

$$\text{Molarity} = \frac{\text{Weight of Benzoic acid (g)}}{122 \times \text{Volume of sod. methoxide used (L)}} \times 100$$

where, 122 is the molecular weight of benzoic acid

2. Determination of ethosuximide

Weight of sample = (W) g

The volume of 0.1M $HClO_4$ consumed = V mL

141.17 g $C_7H_{11}NO_2$ (Ethosuximide)

Each mL of 0.1M perchloric acid solution = 0.0141 g $C_7H_{11}NO_2$

The % of ethosuximide present in the sample is given by:

$$\% \text{ of Ethosuximide} = \frac{0.0141 \times V \times \text{Molarity (cal.)}}{\text{Molarity (given)} \times W} \times 100$$

CHAPTER 6

Complexometric Titrations

Introduction

The technique involves titrating metal ions with a complexing agent or chelating agent (Ligand) and is commonly referred to as complexometric titration. This method represents the analytical application of a complexation reaction. In this method, a simple ion is transformed into a complex ion and the equivalence point is determined by using metal indicators or electrometrically. Various other names such as chilometric titrations, chilometry and EDTA titrations have been used to describe this method. All these terms refer to same analytical method and they have resulted from the use of EDTA (Ethylene diamine tetra acetic acid) and other chilons. These chilons react with metal ions to form a special type of complex known as chelate.

$$\text{Metal ion + Complexing agent} \xrightarrow{\text{Metal-ion Indicators}} \text{Chelate}$$

The molecules or ions which displace the solvent molecules are called **Ligands**. Ligands or complexing agents or chelating agents can be any electron donating entity, which has the ability to bind to the metal ion and produce a complex ion. Ligands having more than one electron donating groups are called **chelating agents**. The most effective complexing agent in ligands are amino and carboxylate ions.

As a sequestering agent, ethylenediaminetetra-acetic acid reacts with most polyvalent metal ions to form water-soluble complexes which cannot be extracted from aqueous solutions with organic solvents. EDTA forms chelates with nearly all metal ions and this reaction is the basis for general analytical method for these ions by titration with a standard EDTA solution. Such titrations are called **complexometric or EDTA titrations**.

Disodium salt of EDTA is a water soluble chelating agent and is always preferred. It is non-hygroscopic and a very stable sequestering agent (Ligands which form water soluble chelates are called sequestering agents). EDTA and 8-hydroxy quinoline are important reagents used in analytical chemistry. Sequestering agents are used to liberate or solubilize metal ions. The agents which form water insoluble chelates are used to remove the metal ions from solution by precipitation.

EDTA has the widest general application in analysis because of the following important properties:

- It has low cost.

- The special structure of its anion which has 6 ligand atoms.

- It forms strainless five-membered rings.

End point in complexometric titration can be detected by indicators. Various indicators used in these titrations are given below in Table:

S. No.	Name of the indicator	Color change	pH range	Metals detected
1.	Mordant black II	Red to blue	6-7	Ca, Ba, Mg, Zn, Cd, Mn, Pb, Hg
	Erichrome black T			
	Solochrome black T			
2.	Murexide or ammonium purpurate	Violet to blue	12	Ca, Cu, Co
3.	Catechol-violet	Violet to red	8-10	Mn, Mg, Fe, Co, Pb
4.	Methyl blue	Blue to yellow	4-5	Pb, Zn, Cd, Hg
	Thymol bue	Blue to grey	10-12	
5.	Alizarin	Red to yellow	4.3	Pb, Zn, Co, Mg, Cu
6.	Sodium Alizarin sulphonate	Blue to red	4	Al, Throium
7.	Xylenol range	Lemon to yellow	1-3	Bi, Thorium
			4-5	Pb, Zn
			5-6	Cd, Hg

Experiment 6.1

To Prepare and Standardize 0.05M Disodium EDTA

Theory

Many metal ions react with electron pair donors to form coordination compounds or complex ions. The formation of a particular class of coordination compounds, called chelates, are especially well suited for quantitative methods. A chelate is formed when a metal ion coordinates with two (or more) donor groups of a single ligand. Tertiary amine compounds such as ethylenediaminetetraacetic acid (EDTA) is widely used for the formation of chelates.

Chemical reaction

$$Zn + 2HCl \longrightarrow ZnCl_2 + H_2$$

$$ZnCl_2 + C_{10}H_{14}N_2Na_2O_8 \longrightarrow C_{10}H_{14}N_2O_8Zn + 2NaCl$$

Chemicals required

1. **0.05M EDTA Solution:** Dissolve accurately weighed 18.6 g of EDTA disodium in distilled water and make up the volume up to 1 liter.

2. Mordant black II

Procedure

1. Weigh accurately 0.8 g of granulated Zinc and transfer to the conical flask.

2. Dissolve it in dilute Hydrochloric acid and 0.1 mL of bromine solution by gentle warming.

3. Boil to remove the excess bromine, cool and add sufficient water to produce 250 mL.

4. Pipette 20 mL in to a conical flask and nearly neutralize with 2M sodium hydroxide.

5. Add about 125 mL water and sufficient ammonia buffer pH 10 to dissolve the precipitates and add 5 mL in excess.

6. Add 50 mg of mordant black II mixture and titrate with the prepared disodium edentate solution until the solution turns to green point.

7. Each mL of 0.5M disodium edetate solution = 0.00327 g of Zinc

Note:

(a) Discard the solution after 30 days.

(b) Restandardize before use.

(c) Store in amber bottle with well fitted suitable stoppers which prevents access to atmospheric carbon dioxide. Standardization can also be done by titration against $CaCO_3$ or ZnO using appropriate metallic indicator.

Observation and Calculations

Standardization of EDTA solution

$$\text{Molarity} = \frac{W(g) \times 20}{250 \times 327 \times V}$$

where,   W = weight of zinc in g.

V = Volume of EDTA consumed (in liter).

327 is the molecular weight of EDTA salt

Experiment 6.2

To Perform Assay of Magnesium Sulphate I.P.

Theory

Magnesium sulfate is commercially available as heptahydrate, monohydrate, anhydrous or dried form containing the equivalent of 2-3 waters of hydration. Magnesium sulfate occurs naturally in seawater, minerals springs and in minerals such as kieserite and epsomite. Magnesium sulfate heptahydrate is manufactured by dissolution of kieserite in water and subsequent crystallization of the heptahydrate. Complexometric titrations with EDTA have been reported for the analysis of nearly all metal ions. Because EDTA has four acidic protons the formation of metal-ion/EDTA complexes is dependent upon the pH. For the titration of Mg^{2+}, one must buffer the solution to a pH of 10 so that complex formation will be quantitative. The reaction of Mg^{2+} with EDTA may be expressed as:

$$Mg^{2+} + H^2Y^{2-} = MgY^{2-} + 2H^+$$

The endpoint of the titration is determined by the addition of Eriochrome Black T, which forms a colored chelate with Mg^{2+} and undergoes a color change when the Mg^{2+} is released to form a chelate with EDTA.

Chemicals required

1. **0.05M EDTA Solution:** Dissolve accurately weighed 18.6 g of EDTA disodium in distilled water and make up the volume to 1 liter.

2. **Ammonia buffer solution:** Dissolve 70 g of NH_4Cl and add 568 mL of conc. Ammonia solution and dilute with distilled water to 1 liter.

3. **Erichrome Black T indicator (EBT):** Dissolve 0.5 g of the dye in 100 mL of rectified spirit.

Procedure

1. Standardization of 0.05M Disodium EDTA solution

(i)   Weigh accurately about 0.8 g of Granulated Zinc and transfer to the conical flask.

(ii)   Dissolve it in dilute Hydrochloric acid and 0.1 mL of bromine solution by gentle warming.

(iii)   Boil to remove the excess bromine, cool and add sufficient water to produce 250 mL.

(iv)   Pipette 20 mL in to a conical flask and nearly neutralize with 2M sodium hydroxide.

(v)   Add about 125 mL water and sufficient ammonia buffer pH 10 to dissolve the precipitates and add 5 mL in excess.

(vi)   Add 50 mg of mordant black II mixture and titrate with the prepared disodium edentate solution until the solution turns to green point.

(vii)   Each mL of 0.5M disodium edetate solution = 0.00327 g of Zinc

2. Determination of Magnesium sulfate

(i)   Accurately weigh about 0.5 g of the ignited sample, dissolve in 5 mL of hydrochloric acid TS, dilute with water to 100 mL, and mix.

(ii)   Transfer 50 mL of this solution into a 250 mL conical flask; add 10 mL of ammonia/ammonium chloride buffer TS and 0.1 mL of Eriochrome Black T indicator.

(iii)   Titrate with 0.05M Disodium EDTA until the color of red-purple solution changes to blue.

(iv)   Perform a blank titration.

Observation and Calculations

1. Standardization of EDTA solution

$$\text{Molarity} = \frac{W(g) \times 20}{250 \times 327 \times V}$$

where,   W = weight of zinc in g.

V = Volume of EDTA consumed (in liter).

327 is the molecular weight of EDTA salt

2. Determination of Magnesium sulfate

Molecular weight of $MgSO_4$ = 120.39

Weight of sample = W g

The volume of 0.05M EDTA consumed in titration of the sample = V_1 mL

The volume of 0.05M EDTA consumed in blank titration = V_2 mL

Difference = $V_1 - V_2$ = V mL

$MgSO_4 = Mg^{2+} = C_{10}H_{14}N_2Na_2O_8$

120.39 g $MgSO_4$ = 1000 mL of M $C_{10}H_{14}N_2Na_2O_8$ solution

Each mL of 0.05M EDTA solution = 0.006019 g of $MgSO_4$

$$\% \text{ purity of } MgSO_4 = \frac{0.006019 \times V \times \text{Molarity (cal.)}}{W \times 0.05 \text{ (molarity given)}} \times 100$$

Experiment 6.3

To Perform Assay of Calcium Chloride

Theory

It occurs as white deliquescent odorless crystals or granules, having slight bitter taste. It is soluble in water and alcohol. Calcium chloride can be injected as intravenous therapy for the treatment of hypocalcaemia. It can be used for magnesium intoxication. Calcium chloride can be used to quickly treat calcium channel blocker toxicity, due to the side effects of drugs such as diltiazem – attenuating potential heart attacks.

Chemical reaction

$$Ca^{2+} + [H_2X]^{2-} \longrightarrow [CaX]^{2-} + 2H^+$$

$$\text{EDTA}$$

Chemicals required

1. 0.15 g Calcium chloride dihydrate.

2. 3.0 mL Dilute hydrochloric acid (10% w/w of HCl).

3. **0.05M disodium edetate:** Dissolve accurately weighed 18.6 g of EDTA disodium in distilled water and make up the volume to 1 liter.

4. Sodium hydroxide solution (20% w/v in water).

5. 0.1 g Calcon mixture (a mixture of 1 part of calcon with 99 parts of freshly ignited anhydrous Na_2SO_4).

Procedure

1. Standardization of 0.05M Disodium EDTA solution

   (i)   Weigh accurately 0.8 g of Granulated Zinc and transfer to the conical flask.

   (ii) Dissolve it in dilute hydrochloric acid and 0.1 mL of bromine solution by gentle warming.

(iii) Boil to remove the excess bromine, cool and add sufficient water to produce 250 mL.

(iv) Pipette 20 mL in to a conical flask and nearly neutralize with 2m sodium hydroxide.

(v) Add about 125 mL water and sufficient ammonia buffer pH 10 to dissolve the precipitates and add 5 mL in excess.

(vi) Add 50 mg of mordant black II mixture and titrate with the prepared disodium edentate solution until the solution turns to green point.

(vii) Each mL of 0.5M disodium edetate solution = 0.00327 g of Zinc

2. Determination of calcium chloride

(i) Weigh accurately about 0.15 g of calcium chloride dihydrate and transfer it to a conical flask.

(ii) Dissolve it in 50 mL of distilled water.

(iii) Fill the burette with 0.05 M disodium edetate solution up to the mark.

(iv) Titrate the solution in conical flask with 0.05M disodium edetate to within a few ml of the expected end point.

(v) Add 8.0 ml of sodium hydroxide solution and 0.1 g of calcon mixture.

(vi) Continue the titration until the color of the solution changes from pink to a full blue color.

(vii) Each ml of 0.05M disodium edetate is equivalent to 0.007351 g of $CaCl_2. 2H_2O$.

Observation and Calculations

1. Standardization of EDTA soliution

$$\text{Molarity} = \frac{W(g) \times 20}{250 \times 327 \times V}$$

where,   W = weight of zinc in g.

V = Volume of EDTA consumed (in liter).

327 the molecular weight of EDTA salt

2. Determination of Calcium chloride

Molecular weight of $CaCl_2$ = 147.014

Weight of sample = W g

The volume of 0.05M EDTA consumed in titration of the sample = V_1 mL

The volume of 0.05M EDTA consumed in blank titration = V_2 mL

Difference = $V_1 - V_2$ = V mL

$CaCl_2 = Ca^{2+} = C_{10}H_{14}N_2Na_2O_8$

147.014 g $CaCl_2$ = 1000 ml of M $C_{10}H_{14}N_2Na_2O_8$ solution

Each ml of 0.05 M EDTA solution = 0.007351 g of $CaCl_2$

$$\% \text{ purity of } CaCl_2 = \frac{0.007351 \times V \times \text{Molarity (cal.)}}{W \times 0.05 \text{ (molarity given)}} \times 100$$

Experiment 6.4

Determine Percentage Purity of Zinc Sulphate

Theory

Zinc sulfate ($ZnSO_4$) is a colorless crystalline, water-soluble chemical compound. The hydrated form, $ZnSO_4.7H_2O$, the mineral goslarite, was historically known as "white vitriol". It is used as an astringent and emetic. A complexometric titration is a titration in which substance is to be determined is a metal ion in solution. In this experiment, the metal to be determined is Zn^{2+} ion and the complexing agent is EDTA, H_4EDTA. The terminal hydrogen atoms of EDTA are acidic and complete ionization results in the EDTA, $EDTA^{4-}$, the ion complexes with zinc by forming coordinate covalent bonds between Zn^{2+} and two nitrogen atoms and four oxygen atoms.

For the titrated, the solution containing zinc ion is first buffered, then the indicator is added. The indicator immediately forms a wine red complex with zinc ion, $ZnIn^-$. Only about 1% of the total zinc ion concentration is complexed. When the titrant is added, it first forms complex with the free zinc ion forming a colorless $ZnEDTA^{4-}$ ion. When all of the free zinc has been complexed, the $EDTA^{4-}$ will take zinc from the $ZnIn^-$ complex, the $ZnEDTA^{2-}$ complex is stronger. The wine-red of $ZnIn^-$ complex will begin to disappear and blue color of HIn^{2-} will appear.

Chemicals required

1. **0.05M EDTA Solution:** Dissolve accurately weighed 18.6 g of EDTA disodium in distilled water and make up the volume to 1 liter.

2. **Ammonia buffer solution:** Dissolve 70 g of NH_4Cl and add 568 mL of conc. Ammonia solution and dilute with distilled water to 1 liter.

3. **Eriochrome Black T indicator (EBT):** Dissolve 0.5 g of the dye in 100 mL of rectified spirit.

Procedure

1. Standardization of 0.05M disodium EDTA solution

(i)   Weigh accurately 0.8 g of granulated zinc and transfer to the conical flask.

(ii)   Dissolve it in dilute hydrochloric acid and 0.1 mL of bromine solution by gentle warming.

(iii) Boil to remove the excess bromine, cool and add sufficient water to produce 250 mL.

(iv)   Pipette 20 mL in to a conical flask and nearly neutralize with 2 M sodium hydroxide.

(v)   Add about 125 mL water and sufficient ammonia buffer of pH 10 to dissolve the precipitates and add 5 mL in excess.

(vi)   Add 50 mg of mordant black II mixture and titrate with the prepared disodium edentate solution until the solution turns to green point.

(vii) Each mL of 0.5M disodium edetate solution = 0.00327 g of Zinc.

2. Determination of Zinc sulfate

(i)   Accurately weigh about 0.3 g of the ignited sample, dissolve in 100 mL of water.

(ii)   Add 5 ml of ammonia/ ammonium chloride buffer TS and 0.1 mL of Eriochrome Black T indicator.

(iii) Titrate with 0.05 M Disodium EDTA until the color of red-purple solution changes to deep blue.

(iv)   Perform a blank titration.

Observation and Calculations

1. Standardization of EDTA solution

$$\text{Molarity} = \frac{W(g) \times 20}{250 \times 327 \times V}$$

where,   W = weight of zinc in g.

V = Volume of EDTA consumed (in liter).

327 the molecular weight of EDTA salt.

2. Determination of Zinc sulfate

Weight of sample = W g

The volume of 0.05M EDTA consumed in titration of sample = V_1 mL

The volume of 0.05M EDTA consumed in blank titration = V_2 mL

Difference = $V_1 V_2 = V$ mL

$ZnSO_4 = Zn^{2+} = C_{10}H_{14}N_2Na_2O_8$

Each ml of 0.05 M EDTA solution = 0.01438 g of $ZnSO_4. 7H_2O$

$$\% \text{ purity of } ZnSO_4 = \frac{0.01438 \times V \times \text{Molarity (cal.)}}{W \times 0.05 \text{ (molarity given)}} \times 100$$

Experiment 6.5

To Determine Percentage Purity of Calcium Gluconate

Theory

It exists as odorless white crystalline granules or powder. Its 1 g is soluble in 30 mL of water; 5 mL of boiling water and insoluble in alcohol, chloroform and ether. 10% calcium gluconate solution (given intravenously) is the form of calcium most widely used in the treatment of hypocalcemia. It is assayed by direct complexometric method. As it is less soluble in water, it is dissolved in boiling water and then cooled. The pH (about 10) is adjusted with ammonia-ammonium chloride buffer. Calcium ions form a stable complex with EDTA disodium (Na_2H_4Y) salt.

Chemical reaction

$$Na_2H_2Y^{2-} + Ca^{2+} \longrightarrow Na_2CaY^{2-} + 2H^+$$

Main reaction

$$Na_2H_2Y^{2-} + Mg^{2+} \longrightarrow Na_2MgY^{2-} + 2H^+$$

At end point

$$Na_2H_2Y^{2-} + MgIn^- \longrightarrow Na_2MgY^{2-} + HIn^{2-} + H^+$$

$$\underset{\substack{\textbf{Wine} \\ \textbf{red}}}{\phantom{Na_2H_2Y^{2-} + MgIn^-}} \qquad\qquad \underset{\substack{\textbf{Sky} \\ \textbf{blue}}}{\phantom{Na_2MgY^{2-} + HIn^{2-} + H^+}}$$

Chemicals required

1. Calcium gluconate

2. **0.05M disodium edetate:** Dissolve accurately weighed 18.6 g of EDTA disodium in distilled water and make up the volume to 1 liter.

3. Dilute hydrochloric acid

4. **Ammonia-ammonium chloride buffer:** Dissolve 70 g of NH_4Cl and add 568 mL of conc. Ammonia solution and dilute with distilled water to 1 liter.

5. **0.05M magnesium sulphate solution:** Dissolve 6.1 g of magnesium sulphate in distilled water and make up the volume up to 1 liter.

6. Mordant black II indicator

Procedure

1. **Standardization of 0.05M Disodium EDTA solution**

    (i)   Weigh accurately about 0.8 g of granulated zinc and transfer to the conical flask.

    (ii)   Dissolve it in dilute hydrochloric acid and 0.1 mL of bromine solution by gentle warming.

    (iii) Boil to remove the excess bromine, cool and add sufficient water to produce 250 mL.

    (iv)   Pipette 20 mL in to a conical flask and nearly neutralize with 2M sodium hydroxide.

    (v)   Add about 125 mL water and sufficient ammonia buffer pH 10 to dissolve the precipitates and add 5 mL in excess.

    (vi)   Add 50 mg of mordant black II mixture and titrate with the prepared disodium edentate solution until the solution turns to green point.

    (vii) Each mL of 0.5M disodium edetate solution = 0.00327 g of Zinc.

2. **Determination of calcium gluconate**

    (i)   Weigh accurately 0.8 g of calcium gluconate.

    (ii)   Dissolve it in 150 mL of water containing 5 mL of dilute hydrochloric acid.

    (iii) Add 15 mL of ammonia-ammonium chloride buffer and 40 mg of mordant black II indicator.

    (iv)   Add 5 mL of 0.05M magnesium sulphate in order to make the end point sharp.

    (v)   Titrate the above solution with standardized 0.05M sodium edetate solution until the solution is deep blue in color.

Observation and Calculations

1. Standardization of EDTA solution

$$\text{Molarity} = \frac{W(g) \times 20}{250 \times 327 \times V}$$

where, W = weight of zinc in g.

   V = Volume of EDTA consumed (in liter).

   327 the molecular weight of EDTA salt.

2. Determination of Calcium gluconate

Weight of sample = W g

The volume of 0.05M EDTA consumed in titration of sample

$= V_2$ mL

The volume of 0.05 M EDTA consumed in blank titration = V_2 mL

Difference = $V_1 - V_2 = V$ mL

Each ml of 0.05 M EDTA solution = 0.02242 g of calcium gluconate

$$\% \text{ purity of calcium gluconate} = \frac{0.02242 \times V \times \text{Molarity (cal.)}}{W \times 0.05 \ (\text{molarity given})} \times 100$$

Experiment 6.6

To Determine Percentage Purity of Potassium Aluminium Sulphate

Theory

Potassium aluminium sulphate, commonly known as Potassium alum, is an astringent/styptic and antiseptic. It can also be used as a natural deodorant by inhibiting the growth of bacteria responsible for body odor. The solution of potassium alum is heated with an excess of disodium edetate to ensure complete formation of aluminium-edetate complex. Hexamine serves as a buffer thereby stabilizing the pH between 5 and 6, (the ideal pH for the titration of the disodium edentate) not required by the Al with 0.05M lead nitrate employing xylenol orange as indicator.

Chemical reaction

$$Al^{3+} + [H_2X]^{2-} \longrightarrow [AlX]^- + 2H^+$$

Chemicals required

1. 1.7 g Potassium alum.

2. **0.05M disodium edetate:** Dissolve accurately weighed 18.6 g of EDTA disodium in distilled water and make up the volume to 1 liter.

3. 1.0 g hexamine.

4. **0.05M lead nitrate:** Dissolve 16.56 g of lead nitrate in 1 liter of distilled water.

5. 0.4 mL xylenol orange solution (0.1% w/v in water).

Procedure

1. **Standardization of 0.05M Disodium EDTA solution**

    (i) Weigh accurately about 0.8 g of Granulated Zinc and transfer to the conical flask.

    (ii) Dissolve it in dilute hydrochloric acid and 0.1 mL of bromine solution by gentle warming.

(iii) Boil to remove the excess bromine, cool and add sufficient water to produce 250 mL.

(iv) Pipette 20 mL in to a conical flask and nearly neutralize with 2M sodium hydroxide.

(v) Add about 125 mL water and sufficient ammonia buffer pH 10 to dissolve the precipitates and add 5 mL in excess.

(vi) Add 50 mg of mordant black II mixture and titrate with the prepared disodium edentate solution until the solution turns to green point.

(vii) Each mL of 0.5M disodium edetate solution = 0.00327 g of Zinc.

2. Determination of purity of potassium aluminium sulphate:

(i) Weigh accurately 1.7 g of potassium aluminium and dissolve it in 50 mL distilled water in a conical flask.

(ii) Add 50 mL of 0.05M disodium edetate.

(iii) Heat the contents of flask over a water-bath for 10 minutes to allow completion of complexation and cool to ambient temperature.

(iv) Now, add 1 g hexamine to act as buffer and titrate excess sodium edetate with 0.05 M lead nitrate employing 0.4 mL of xylenol orange solution as an indicator.

(v) The color will change from that of the indicator (yellow at the pH of the titration) to the corresponding reddish purple, the color of the lead complex of the indicator.

(vi) Each ml of 0.05M disodium edetate is equivalent to 0.02372 g of $KAl(SO_4)_2$, $12H_2O$.

Observation and Calculations

1. Standardization of EDTA solution

$$\text{Molarity} = \frac{W(g) \times 20}{250 \times 327 \times V}$$

where,   W = weight of zinc in g.

V = Volume of EDTA consumed (in liter).

327 the molecular weight of EDTA salt.

2. Determination of Potassium aluminium sulphate

Weight of sample = W g

The volume of 0.05 M EDTA added = V_1 mL

The volume of 0.05 M lead nitrate consumed in back titration = V_2 mL

The volume of 0.05 M EDTA consumed in titration of sample = $V_1 - V_2 = V$ mL

Each mL of 0.05M EDTA solution = 0.02372 g of potassium aluminium sulphate

% purity of potassium aluminium sulphate =

$$\frac{0.02372 \times V \times \text{Molarity (cal.)}}{W \times 0.05 \ (\text{molarity given})} \times 100$$

Experiment 6.7

To Determine Percentage Purity of Sodium Chloride

Theory

Sodium chloride, also known as **salt, common salt, table salt** or **halite**, is an ionic compound with the formula NaCl. Sodium chloride is used in veterinary medicine as emesis causing agent. It is given as warm saturated solution.

Chemical equation

$$AgNO_3 + NaCl \longrightarrow AgCl + NaNO_3$$

Chemicals required

1. **0.1M Silver nitrate solution (AgNO₃):** Prepared by dissolving 1.7 g of silver nitrate in 100 mL in distilled water.

2. **0.1M sodium chloride (NaCl) solution:** Prepared by dissolving 2.922 g in 500 mL of distilled water.

3. Sodium chloride.

4. Potassium chromate solution (5% w/v in water).

Procedure

1. **Standardization of silver nitrate solution**

   (i)   Pipette out 10 mL of 0.1M NaCl solution in a clean flask.

   (ii) Add 1 mL of potassium chromate indicator.

   (iii) Titrate the content of the flask against 0.1M AgNO₃ solution until brick red colored precipitate is formed.

   (iv) Repeat the titration to get three concordant readings

   (v)   Calculate the normality of AgNO₃ used.

2. Determine purity of sodium chloride

   (i)   Weigh accurately 0.25 g of sodium chloride and transfer it in a conical flask.

  (ii) Dissolve it in 50 mL of distilled water.

 (iii) Titrate the solution in conical flask with 0.1N silver nitrate solution.

 (iv) Add 2-3 drops of potassium chromate solution as indicator.

  (v) Continue the titration until the end point from yellow to brick red color is indicated.

 (vi) Each mL of 0.1N silver nitrate solution is equivalent to 0.007455 g of NaCl.

Observation and Calculations

1. Standardization of silver nitrate solution

$$\text{Molarity of AgNO}_3 = \frac{W}{58.44 \times V\,(\text{in liter})}$$

where,   W = weight of sodium chloride in g

           V = volume of silver nitrate solution consumed in liter

           58.44 molecular weight of sodium chloride

2. Determination of Sodium chloride

Weight of sample = W g

The volume of 0.1M silver nitrate added = V mL

Each mL of 0.1M silver nitrate = 0.007455 g of sodium chloride

% of sodium chloride =

$$\frac{0.007455 \times \text{vol. of silver nitrate used} \times \text{molarity}\,(\text{cal.}) \times 100}{\text{Weight of the sample}\,(\text{g}) \times 0.1\,(\text{molarity given})}$$

Experiment 6.8

To Determine Percentage Purity of Ammonium Chloride

Theory

An aqueous solution of ammonium chloride is slightly acidic, the end point is indistinct when titrated directly with silver nitrate ($AgNO_3$) solution. Therefore, Volhard's method is adopted which is explained as follows: Ammonium thiocyanate solution is used along with N/10 $AgNO_3$ solution for the estimation of the substances which reacts with $AgNO_3$ but which cannot be determined by direct titration with $AgNO_3$. Excess amount of standard $AgNO_3$ solution is added together with concentrated HNO_3, and the excess $AgNO_3$ titrated with N/10 NH_4 SCN solution.

Chemical reaction

$$NH_4Cl + AgNO_3 \longrightarrow AgCl + NH_4NO_3$$

Ammonium **Silver**   **Silver**
chloride   **nitrate**   **chloride**

$$AgNO_3 + NH_4SCN \longrightarrow AgSCN + NH_4NO_3$$

Ammonium   **Silver**
thiocyanate   **thiocyanate**

Chemicals required

1. **0.1M Silver nitrate solution ($AgNO_3$):** Prepared by dissolving 1.7 g of silver nitrate in 100 mL in distilled water.

2. **0.1M sodium chloride (NaCl) solution:** Prepared by dissolving 2.922 g in 500 mL of distilled water.

3. Ammonium chloride.

4. Concentrated nitric acid.

5. Nitrobenzene.

6. Ferric ammonium sulphate indicator

7. **0.1M ammonium thiocyanate (NH₄SCN) solution:** prepared by dissolving 0.76 g ammonium thiocyanate in 100 mL in distilled water.

Procedure

1. **Standardization of silver nitrate solution**

    (i)   Pipette out 10 mL of 0.1M NaCl solution in a clean flask.

    (ii) Add 1mL of potassium chromate indicator.

    (iii) Titrate the content of the flask against 0.1M $AgNO_3$ solution until brick red colored precipitates are formed.

    (iv) Repeat the titration to get three concordant readings

    (v)   Calculate the normality of $AgNO_3$ used.

2. **Determine purity of ammonium chloride**

    (i)   Weigh accurately 0.2 g of the sample and dissolve in 35 mL distilled water.

    (ii) Add 15 mL HNO_3 and 5 mL nitrobenzene and 50 mL 0.1 M silver nitrate.

    (iii) Shake the mixture vigorously for 1 minute.

    (iv) Add 5 mL of ferric ammonium sulphate indicator and titrate with 0.1 M ammonium thiocyanate (NH₄SCN) solution to the reddish-brown color as the end point.

Observation and Calculations

1. **Standardization of silver nitrate solution**

$$\text{Molarity of } AgNO_3 = \frac{W}{58.44 \times V\,(\text{in liter})}$$

where,   W = weight of sodium chloride in g

             V = volume of silver nitrate solution consumed in liter

             58.44 molecular weight of sodium chloride

2. **Determination of Ammonium chloride**

Weight of sample = W g

The volume of 0.1M silver nitrate added = V_1 mL

The volume of 0.1M ammonium thiocyanate consumed in back titration = V_2 mL

The volume of 0.1M silver nitrate consumed in titration of sample = $V_1 - V_2 = V$ mL

Each ml of 0.1M silver nitrate = 0.05349 g of ammonium chloride

% of ammonium chloride =

$$\frac{0.005349 \times \text{vol. of silver nitrate used} \times \text{molarity (cal.)} \times 100}{\text{Weight of the sample(g)} \times 0.1 \ (\text{molarity given})}$$

CHAPTER 7

Kjeldahl Titration

The Kjeldahl method was developed in 1883 by a brewer called Johann Kjeldahl. The method is applicable to the determination of nitrogen occurring in the tri-negative state in food and raw materials. The method consists of three steps: digestion, distillation and titration.

Digestion

The sample to be analyzed is weighed into a *digestion flask* and then digested by heating it in the presence of sulfuric acid (an oxidizing agent which digests the sample), anhydrous sodium sulfate (to speed up the reaction by raising the boiling point) and a catalyst, such as copper, selenium, titanium, or mercury (to speed up the reaction). Digestion converts any nitrogen in the sample (other than that form of nitrates or nitrites) into ammonia, and other organic matter to CO_2 and H_2O. Ammonia gas is not liberated in an acid solution because the ammonia is in the form of the ammonium ion (NH_4^+) which binds to the sulfate ion (SO_4^{2-}) and thus remains in solution:

$$\text{Organic (N)} + H_2SO_4 \longrightarrow (NH_4)SO_4 + CO_2 + H_2O$$

Distillation

After the digestion has been completed, the digestion flask is connected to a *receiving flask* by a tube. The solution in the digestion flask is then made alkaline by addition of sodium hydroxide, which converts the ammonium sulfate into ammonia gas:

$$(NH_4)_2SO_4 + 2NaOH \longrightarrow 2NH_3 + 2H_2O + Na_2SO_4$$

The ammonia gas that is formed is liberated from the solution and moves out of the digestion flask and into the receiving flask, which contains an excess of boric acid. The low pH of the solution in the receiving flask converts the ammonia gas into the ammonium ion.

Titration

Titration quantifies the amount of ammonia in the receiving solution. The amount of nitrogen in a sample can be calculated from the quantified amount of ammonium ion in the receiving solution. There are two types of titrations: back and direct titration. Both methods indicate the ammonia present in the distillate with a color change.

Advantages and Disadvantages of Kjeldahl method

Advantages

(a) The Kjeldahl method is most widely used and still considered as the standard method for comparison against all other methods.

(b) Its universality, high precision and good reproducibility have made it the primary method for the estimation of protein in foods.

Disadvantages

(a) It does not give a measure of the true protein, since all nitrogen in foods is not in the form of protein.

(b) Different proteins need different correction factors because they have different amino acid sequences.

(c) The use of concentrated sulfuric acid at high temperatures poses a considerable hazard, as does the use of some of the possible catalysts.

(d) The technique is time consuming.

Experiment 7.1

To Determine Nitrogen Content in a given Sample

Theory

The method consists of heating a substance with sulfuric acid which decomposes the organic nitrogen present to ammonium sulfate. In this step potassium sulfate is added in order to increase the boiling point of the medium (from 337 °C to 373 °C). Chemical composition of the sample is complete when the medium has become clear colorless (initially very dark). Potassium sulfate (K_2SO_4) (also known as potash of sulfur) is a non-flammable white crystalline salt which is soluble in water.

The solution is then distilled with sodium hydroxide (added in small quantities) which converts the ammonium salt to ammonia. The amount of ammonia present in (hence the amount of nitrogen present in the sample) is determined by back titration. The end of the condenser is dipped into a solution of hydrochloric acid or sulfuric acid of precisely known concentration. The ammonia reacts with the acid and the remainder of the acid is then titrated with standard sodium hydroxide solution with a phenolphthalein pH indicator.

Chemical equation

$$Protein + H_2SO_4 \longrightarrow CO_2 + (NH_4)_2SO_4 + SO_2$$

$$(NH_4)_2SO_4 + 2NaOH \longrightarrow Na_2SO_4 + NH_4OH$$

$$2NH_4OH + H_2SO_4 \longrightarrow (NH_4)_2SO_4 + 2H_2O$$

Chemicals required

1. Sulfuric acid, concentrated, 95-98 %, reagent grade.
2. 0.1N Sodium hydroxide solution.
3. Potassium sulfate (K_2SO_4).

4. Anhydrous Copper sulfate ($CuSO_4$).

5. 0.5N hydrochloric acid. Prepare by diluting 43.0 mL 36.5 to 38% HCl to 0.1 liter with distilled water.

Procedure

A. Digestion

1. Weigh approximately 1 g of powdered sample into digestion flask, recording weight (W) to nearest 0.1 mg. Include reagent blank and highly purity lysine HCl as check of correctness of digestion parameters.

2. Add 15 g of potassium sulfate, 0.04 g anhydrous copper sulfate, 0.5 to 1.0 g alundum granules, or add 16.7 g K_2SO_4, 0.01 g anhydrous copper sulfate, 0.6 g TiO_2 and 0.3 g pumice. Then, add 20 mL sulfuric acid (add additional 1.0 mL sulfuric acid for each 0.1 g fat or 0.2 g other organic matter if sample weight is greater than 1 g).

3. Heat samples on the digestion unit (heater setting 5-7) while aspirating.

4. With a hot glove and tongs, rotate flasks occasionally to prevent sticking and to expose all surfaces to acid.

5. Heat until samples is clear (this may take 30-45 min.). Some samples will be clear with a slight color pigment.

6. When complete, cool the flasks for 5-10 min.

7. Add 10 mL of de-ionized water to the cooled digestion flask for transferring to the distillation unit.

B. Distillation

1. Prepare titration flask by adding appropriate volume of accurately measured standard HCl solution to amount of water so that condenser tip is immersed (try 15 mL acid and 70 mL water if undecided).

2. For reagent blank, pipette 1 mL of acid and add approximately 85 mL water. Add 3 to 4 drops methyl red indicator solution.

3. Add 2 to 3 drops of tri-butyl citrate or other antifoam agent to digestion flask to reduce foaming.

4. Slowly transfer the content to distillation flask, add sufficient 45% sodium hydroxide solution (approximatcly 80 mL) to make mixture strongly alkaline.

5. Heat to distill out ammonia which is collected in titration flask containing hydrochloric acid.

6. Remove the titration flask from unit, rinsing the condenser tube with distilled water as the flask is being removed.

C. Titration

Titrate excess acid with standard sodium hydroxide solution to orange end point (color change from red to orange to yellow) and record volume to nearest 0.01 mL. Titrate the reagent blank similarly.

Observation and Calculations

For percent nitrogen

Mass of the organic compound = W g

Vol. of the acid required for complete neutralization of the evolved ammonia = V mL

Normality of the standard HCl = N

From the law of equivalence (normality equation),

Then V mL of N acid = V mL of NH_3

NV milli equivalent of acid = NV milli equivalent of ammonia

Therefore,

$$\text{Mass of nitrogen in the evolved ammonia} = \frac{14 \times N \times V}{1000}\, g$$

$$\% \text{ of nitrogen in the sample} = \frac{14 \times N \times V}{1000} \times \frac{100}{W} \times \frac{1.4\,NV}{W}$$

CHAPTER 8

Karl-Fischer Titration

A plethora of chemical compounds for the determination of small amounts of water present in organic solids, pharmaceutical substances and organic solvents have been devised over a length of time. But unquestionably the most important of these is the one proposed by Karl Fischer (1935), which is considered to be relatively specific for water. The titrimetric determination of water by the Karl Fischer method depends on the reaction that takes place quantitatively between water and a reagent consisting of sulfur dioxide and iodine in anhydrous pyridine and usually methanol. The reaction is carried out in a suitable solvent such as methanol or acetic acid. The reagents and solutions used in the determination of water by this method are sensitive to water and precautions must be taken throughout to prevent exposure to atmospheric moisture.

The titration vessel is fitted with two platinum electrodes, a gas inlet tube if needed, a stopper, which accommodates the burette tip, and a vent tube protected by a desiccant. The substance to be titrated is introduced through an inlet tube or side-arm, which can be closed by an airtight stopper. The Karl Fischer reagent TS is protected from light and stored in a bottle into which is fitted an automatic burette. The reagent is pumped into the burette by means of a hand bellows, the access of moisture being prevented by a suitable arrangement of desiccant tubes. Stirring is accomplished magnetically or by means of a stream of suitably dried nitrogen passed through the solution during the titration.

The end-point is obtained by using an electrical circuit composed of a microammeter, platinum electrodes, and a 1.5 V or 2 V battery connected across a variable resistance of about 2000 Ω. The resistance is adjusted so that an initial current passes through the platinum electrodes in series with a microammeter. After each addition of reagent, the pointer of the microammeter is deflected but quickly returns to its original position. At the end of the reaction a deflection is obtained that persists for 10-15 seconds. Alternatively, the end-point can also be determined by a voltametric method. A potential difference of 30-50 mV is applied to the platinum electrodes to serve as a constant polarizing current and the solution is titrated with the reagent. The potential difference is monitored by means of a microvoltmeter. The end-point is reached when the voltmeter indicates a stable decrease of voltage. In the voltametric method the end-point may also be obtained graphically by plotting the voltage versus the volume of the reagent, and establishing the beginning of the drop in potential.

Experiment 8.1

To Determine Moisture Content of Amoxicillin Trihydrate

Theory

A dehydrating solvent suitable for the sample is placed in a flask. Titrant is used to remove all moisture from the solvent. The sample is then added. Titration is carried out using a titrant, the Titer (mg H_2O/mL) of which has previously been determined. The moisture content of the sample is determined from the titration volume (mL). The end point is detected using the constant-current polarization voltage method.

Procedure

1. Accurately weight about 50 mg of water and titrate with Karl Fischer reagent till end point. Note the titre value (V_1 mL).

2. Transfer sufficient dried methanol in a titration vessel and titrate with Karl Fischer reagent till the end.

3. Accurately weigh about 0.6 g of amoxicillin trihydrate and dissolve into the above methanol with stirring. Titrate with Karl Fischer reagent till the end point. Note the titre value (V_1 mL).

Observation and Calculations

Weight of water = W g

Weight of amoxicillin trihydrate = W_1 g

Volume of KF reagent required to titrate water for standardization = V_1 ml

Volume of KF reagent required to titrate amoxicillin trihydrate = V_2 mL

$$\% \text{ of moisture content} = \frac{W \times V_2}{V_1 \times W_1} \times 100$$

Experiment 8.2

To Determine Moisture Content of Prednisolone Sodium Phosphate

Theory

Prednisolone sodium phosphate belongs to the family of medications called *corticosteroids* and is used for its ability to **reduce inflammation in many parts of the body.**

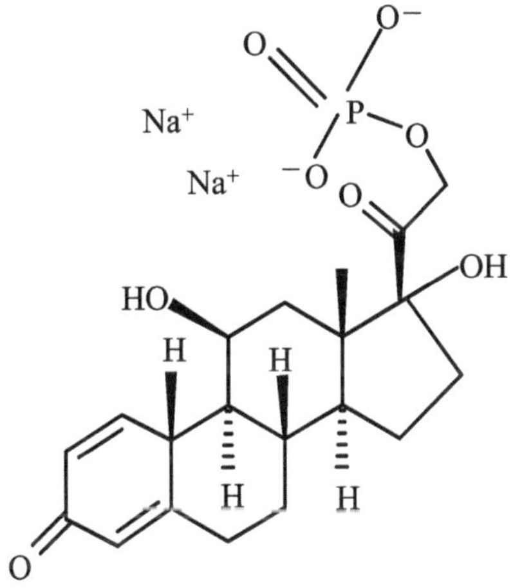

Procedure

1. Accurately weight about 50 mg of water and titrate with Karl Fischer reagent till end point. Note the titre value (V_1 mL).

2. Transfer sufficient dried methanol in a titration vessel and titrate with Karl Fischer reagent till the end.

3. Accurately weigh about 0.6 g of prednisolone sodium phosphate and dissolve into the above methanol with stirring. Titrate with Karl Fischer reagent till the end point. Note the titre value (V_1 mL).

Observation and Calculations

Weight of water = W g

Weight of amoxicillin trihydrate = W_1 g

Volume of KF reagent required to titrate water for standardization = V_1 mL

Volume of KF reagent required to titrate prednisolone sodium phosphate = V_2 mL

$$\% \text{ of moisture content} = \frac{W \times V_2}{V_1 \times W_1} \times 100$$

CHAPTER 9

Diazotization Titration

In general, aromatic primary amino moiety (*i.e.*, Ar-NH$_2$), as present in a host of sulphadrugs *viz.*, succinyl sulphathiazole, sulphamethoxazole, sulphaphenazole and other potent pharmaceutical substances, for instance sodium or calcium aminosalicylate, isocarboxazid, primaquine phosphate, procainamide hydrochloride, procaine hydrochloride and dapsone react with sodium nitrite in an acidic medium to yield the corresponding diazonium salts as expressed below :

$$\text{C}_6\text{H}_5\text{—NH}_2 + \text{NaNO}_2 + \text{HCl} \longrightarrow \text{C}_6\text{H}_5\text{—N} {\equiv} \text{N } \overline{\text{Cl}} + \text{NaCl} + \text{H}_2\text{O}$$

It is interesting to observe here that the above reaction is absolutely quantitative under experimental parameters. Nitrous acid is formed by the interaction of sodium nitrite and hydrochloric acid as follows:

$$\text{NaNO}_2 + \text{HCl} \longrightarrow \text{NaCl} + \text{HNO}_2$$

The end-point in the sodium nitrite titration is determined by the liberation of iodine from iodide which may be expressed by the following equations:

$$\text{KI} + \text{HCl} \longrightarrow \text{HI} + \text{KCl}$$

$$2\text{HI} + 2\text{HNO}_2 \longrightarrow \text{I}_2 + 2\text{NO} + 2\text{H}_2\text{O}$$

In other words, the small excess of HNO$_2$ present at the end-point can be detected visually by employing either starch-iodide paper or paste as an external indicator. Thus, the liberated iodine reacts with starch to form a blue green color which is a very sensitive reaction. Besides, the end-point may also be accomplished electrometrically by adopting the dead-stop end-point technique, using a pair of platinum electrodes immersed in the titration liquid.

Application of diazotization titration: An important pharmaceutical application of sodium nitrite titration is the analysis of sulphonamides by diazotization of primary aromatic amino group usually present in this class of drugs. Several sulphonamides require the formation of primary amine prior to diazotization step.

Example – phthalylsulphathiazole and succinyl sulphathiazole are first hydrolyzed to give primary aromatic amine and determined by $NaNO_2$ titration method.

Experiment 9.1

To Determine Sulphamethoxazole Content in Co-Trimoxazole Tablets

Theory

It is most often used as part of a synergistic combination with trimethoprim in a 5:1 ratio in co-trimoxazole. Its primary activity is against susceptible forms of *Streptococcus, Staphylococcus aureus, Escherichia coli, Haemophilus influenzae,* and oral anaerobes. It is commonly used to treat urinary tract infections. Sulfonamides are structural analogs and competitive antagonists of para-aminobenzoic acid (PABA). They inhibit normal bacterial utilization of PABA for the synthesis of folic acid, an important metabolite in DNA synthesis. The effects seen are usually bacteriostatic in nature. Folic acid is not synthesized in humans, but is instead a dietary requirement. This allows for the selective toxicity to bacterial cells (or any cell dependent on synthesizing folic acid) over human cells. In this titration sulphamethoxazole is diazotized by nitrous acid, produced *in situ* from the reaction of sodium nitrite and hydrochloric acid. Slightly excess nitrous acid reacts with starch iodide paper to mark blue colored end point.

Chemical equation

$$NaNO_2 \; + \; HCl \longrightarrow \; HNO_2 \; + \; NaCl$$

$$H_2NSO_2{-}C_6H_4{-}NH_2 \; + \; HNO_2 \; + \; NaCl \longrightarrow$$

$$H_2NSO_2{-}C_6H_4{-}N_2Cl \; + \; 2H_2O$$

Chemical required

1. **0.1M sodium nitrite (NaNO₂) solution:** Dissolve 7.5 g sodium nitrite in sufficient water to make 1000 mL.

2. Hydrochloric acid

3. Starch iodide paper

Procedure

1. Standardization of 0.1M sodium nitrite solution:

(i) Weigh accurately about 1 g of sulphanilamide and transfer it to the conical flask.

(ii) Dissolve it in 40 mL of concentrated hydrochloric acid and 100 mL of distilled water.

(iii) Cool the solution to about 5 °C.

(iv) Fill the burette with 0.1M sodium nitrite solution up to the mark.

(v) Titrate the solution in conical flask with 0.1M sodium nitrite solution by dipping the tip of burette well into the solution.

(vi) Continue the titration until immediate blue color appears on placing a drop of sodium nitrite solution on starch iodide paper.

2. Determination of sulphamethoxazole:

(i) Weigh 20 tablets to determine their average weight and powder them.

(ii) Weigh the tablet powder equivalent to 0.5 g of sulpha-methoxazole and dissolve in 60 mL of water and 10 mL hydrochloric acid.

(iii) Cool down the mixture to 10 °C and titrate with standardized 0.1M sodium nitrite solution until the drop of reaction mixture gives blue color with starch iodide paper.

Observation and Calculations

Average weight of tablets = X g

Weight of powder = W g

Amount of 0.1M sodium nitrite solution consumed = V mL

Molecular weight of sulphamethoxazole = 253.3

1 mole of sulphamethoxazole = 1 mole of 1M of sodium nitrite = 1/10 of 0.1M sodium nitrite

Hence 1 mLof 0.1M sodium nitrite solution = 0.02533 g of sulphamethoxazole

The content of sulpharmethoxazole in tablet =

$$\frac{0.02533 \times V \times \text{Molarity (cal.)}}{\text{Molarity (given)} \times W} \times Z \text{ g of sulphamethoxazole}$$

$$\% \text{ content of sulphamethoxazole} = \frac{\text{Practical value}}{\text{Theoretical value}} \times 100$$

Experiment 9.2

To Determine Dapsone Content in Tablet Formulation

Theory

Dapsone (diamino-diphenyl sulfone) is most commonly used antibacterial in combination with rifampicin and clofazimine as multidrug therapy for the treatment of *Mycobacterium leprae* infections (leprosy). As an antibacterial, dapsone inhibits bacterial synthesis of dihydrofolic acid, via competition with para-aminobenzoate for the active site of dihydropteroate synthetase. In this titration sulphamethoxazole is diazotized by nitrous acid, produced *in situ* from the reaction of sodium nitrite and hydrochloric acid. Slightly excess nitrous acid reacts with starch iodide paper to mark blue colored end point.

Chemical equation

$$NaNO_2 + HCl \longrightarrow HNO_2 + NaCl$$

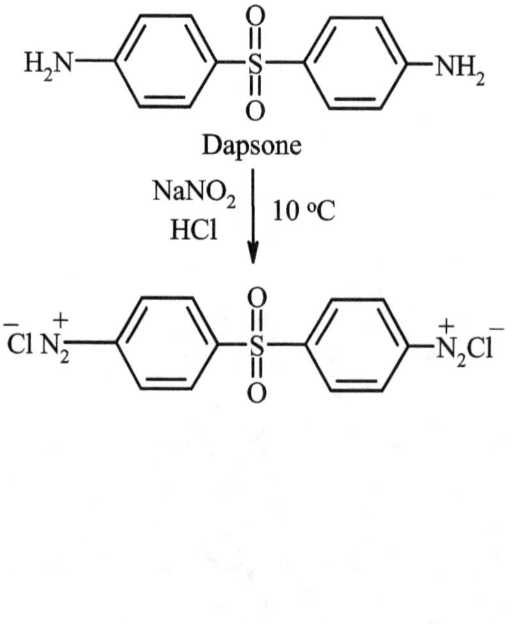

$$H_2N-\!\!\left\langle\bigcirc\right\rangle\!\!-\!\overset{\displaystyle O}{\underset{\displaystyle O}{S}}\!-\!\!\left\langle\bigcirc\right\rangle\!\!-NH_2$$

Dapsone

$$\xrightarrow[HCl]{NaNO_2 \quad 10\ ^{\circ}C}$$

$$Cl^{-}\overset{+}{N_2}-\!\!\left\langle\bigcirc\right\rangle\!\!-\!\overset{\displaystyle O}{\underset{\displaystyle O}{S}}\!-\!\!\left\langle\bigcirc\right\rangle\!\!-\overset{+}{N_2}Cl^{-}$$

Chemicals required

1. **0.1M sodium nitrite (NaNO$_2$) solution:** Dissolve 7.5 g sodium nitrite in sufficient water to make 1000 ml.

2. Hydrochloric acid

3. Starch iodide paper

Procedure

1. Standardization of 0.1M sodium nitrite solution

(i) Weigh accurately 1 g of sulphanilamide and transfer it to the conical flask.

(ii) Dissolve it in 40 mL of concentrated hydrochloric acid and 100 mL of distilled water.

(iii) Cool the solution to about 5 °C.

(iv) Fill the burette with 0.1M sodium nitrite solution up to the mark.

(v) Titrate the solution in conical flask with 0.1M sodium nitrite solution by dipping the tip of burette well into the solution.

(vi) Continue the titration until immediate blue color appears on placing a drop of sodium nitrite solution on starch iodide paper.

2. Determination of dapsone

(i) Weigh 20 tablets to determine their average weight and powder them.

(ii) Weigh the tablet powder equivalent to 0.25 g of dapsone and dissolve in 20 mL of water and 20 mL hydrochloric acid.

(iii) Cool down the mixture to 10 °C and titrate with standardized 0.1 M sodium nitrite solution until the drop of reaction mixture gives blue color with starch iodide paper.

Observation and Calculations

Average weight of tablets = X g

Weight of powder = W g

Amount of 0.1M sodium nitrite solution consumed = V mL

Molecular weight of dapsone = 248.4

1 mole of dapsone = 2 mole of 1M of sodium nitrite = 2000 mL of 1M sodium nitrite

Hence 1 mL of 0.1M sodium nitrite solution = 0.01242 g of dapsone

The content of dapsone in tablet =

$$\frac{0.01242 \times V \times \text{Molarity}\left(\text{cal.}\right)}{\text{Molarity}\left(\text{given}\right) \times W} \times Z \text{ g of dapsone}$$

$$\% \text{ content of dapsone} = \frac{\text{Practical value}}{\text{Theoretical value}} \times 100$$

CHAPTER 10

Conductometric Titrations

Principle of Conductometric Titrations

The principle of conductometric titration is based on the fact that in dilute solutions, ions act independently of each other and they contribute to the conductance of the solution. Both cations and anions have varying degree of conductance. Thus, when a solution of one electrolyte is added to the solution of another electrolyte, the overall conductance depends on whether the reaction takes place or not. If no reaction occurs, the overall conductance of the solution increases. However, when a reaction occurs, replacement/substitution of ions takes place and depending upon the conductance of replacing or replaced ion, overall conductance will increase or decrease.

In conductometric titrations, titrant is added in small volumes and conductivity measured. The points thus obtained after addition of each increment of titrant, is plotted to give a graph which consists of two straight lines intersecting at the equivalence point. Accuracy of the method is greater when the angle of intersecting line is more acute.

Applications of Conductometry:

1. Determination of solubility of sparingly soluble material

2. Kinetic studies based upon the measurement of conductivity before, during and at the end of chemical reaction.

3. The degree of dissociation of weaker electrolytes.

4. To determine the basicity of organic acids.

5. To determine concentration based on the determination of the conductivity of the solution of different concentrations.

Experiment 10.1

To Perform Conductometric Titration of Hydrochloric Acid with Sodium Hydroxide

Theory

Conductance (G) is the reciprocal of electric resistance (R).

$$G = 1/R$$

It is a measure of the ability of a solution to conduct electricity. The conductance of a solution is the sum of the conductances of all of the ions which are in solution. The conductance of a particular ion in solution depends upon the concentration of the ion, the charge on the ion, and the size of the ion. As the concentration or the charge of the ion increases, the conductance of the solution increases. In general as the size of the solvated ion decreases, its mobility through the solution increases and consequently the conductance of the solution increases. In water, H^+, has the greatest conductances. Of the common, negative ions, OH^- has the greatest conductance. Molecular species (uncharged substances) do not contribute to the conductance of the solution. During the titration of hydrochloric acid with sodium hydroxide, the reaction that takes place in the titration vessel is

$$H^+ + Cl^- \xrightarrow{Na^+ \ OH^-} H_2O + Cl^- + Na^+$$

Before the end-point, H^+ is removed from the solution by reaction with OH^-, and Na^+ is added to the solution. Since the relative conductance of H^+ is about seven times of Na^+, the conductance of the solution decreases prior to the end point.

After the end point, no H^+ is available to react, and the conductance of the solution increases as a result of the addition of Na^+ and OH^-. Consequently the titration curve has a V-shaped. The end point of the titration corresponds to the intersection of the extrapolated linear portions of the titration curve.

Conductance is usually measured with an alternating current between two identical, platinized platinum electrodes. Use of an alternating current prevents the buildup of the reaction products around either electrode and consequently prevents polarization of the solution. The electrodes must be rigidly held at a fixed distance apart during the titrations in order to prevent changes in conductance that result from an altered solution volume between the electrodes.

Chemicals required

1. Potassium hydrogen phthalate

2. **Sodium hydroxide:** Prepare 0.1M NaOH solution by dissolving 4 g of NaOH in 1 liter of water.

3. Hydrochloric acid

Procedure

1. Dry potassium hydrogen phthalate at 110 °C in oven for at least 1 hour. After the drying, remove the compound from the oven and allow it cool to room temperature in the desiccator.

2. Weigh between 0.7 and 0.9 g of the cooled potassium hydrogen phthalate into each of three, labeled, 250 mL Erlenmeyer flasks. Record the mass of the solid in each flask.

3. Add 30 mL of distilled or deionized water and two drops of phenolphthalein solution to each flask.

4. Fill the 50 mL burette with the sodium hydroxide solution.

5. Titrate the solution present in each Erlenmeyer flask to the end point with the sodium hydroxide solution.

6. The end point color change is from colorless to light pink. Record the three endpoint volumes to the nearest 0.01 mL.

7. Take at least 35 mL of a hydrochloric acid solution.

8. Use a pipette to add 10 mL of the hydrochloric acid solution to the 250 mL beaker.

9. Add about 140 mL of distilled or deionized water and a stirring bar to the beaker.

10. Place the beaker on a magnetic stirrer.

11. Use a clamp to suspend the electrodes in the solution.

12. The platinum electrodes must be completely submerged in the solution, but they should not interfere with operation of the stirring bar.

13. Adjust the stirring rate to yield a smoothly stirred solution.

14. Refill the burette with sodium hydroxide solution.

15. Measure the initial conductance of the stirred solution.

16. Add 1 mL portions of the sodium and the total volume of the added titrant solution after each addition.

17. Continue the titration until the end point has been passed by 100% i.e., until a total volume that is twice the end-point volume has been added.

18. Similarly dilute and titrate two, more 10 mL portions of the hydrochloric acid solution.

19. After the titrations have been completed, store the electrodes in water.

Observation and Calculations

S. no.	Volume of NaOH	Conductance
1		
2		
3		
4		
5		
6		

1. Use the mass of potassium hydrogen phthalate (M.W. = 204.23) that was in each flask and the corresponding end point volume of the sodium hydroxide solution to calculate three values of the concentration (M) of the sodium hydroxide solution.

2. For each conductometric titration, plot conductance (y axis) as a function of the volume of the added sodium hydroxide solution. Draw a straight line through each of the two, linear portions in each titration curve. Determine the endpoint volume of each titration from the intersection of the two straight lines.

3. Use the endpoint volumes and the mean sodium hydroxide concentration to calculate three values of the concentration of the original hydrochloric acid solution.

Experiment 10.2

To Perform Conductometric Titration of Acetic acid with Sodium Hydroxide

Theory

Since acetic acid is dissociated slightly ($Ka = 1.8 \times 10^{-5}$) in aqueous solution, the conductance of the acetic acid solution is initially less. As sodium hydroxide is added, the hydroxide reacts with the acid to form water and acetate.

$$HC_2H_3O_2 \xrightarrow{\ \ Na^+\ OH^-\ \ } H_2O + Na^+ + C_2H_3O_2^-$$

$$\updownarrow$$

$$H^+ + C_2H_3O_2^-$$

The addition of the $C_2H_3O_2^-$ and Na^+ to the solution causes the conductance of the solution to increase. After the end point, Na^+ and OH^- are added to the solution. Since the relative conductance of OH^- is nearly five times of the $C_2H_3O_2^-$, the conductance of the solution after the end point increases more rapidly than it did before the end point. The end point corresponds to the intersection of the extrapolated linear portions of the curve.

Conductance is usually measured with an alternating current between two identical, platinized platinum electrodes. Use of an alternating current prevents the buildup of the reaction products around either electrode and consequently prevents polarization of the solution. The electrodes must be rigidly held at a fixed distance apart during the titrations in order to prevent changes in conductance that result from an altered solution volume between the electrodes.

Chemicals required

1. Potassium hydrogen phthalate.
2. **Sodium hydroxide:** Prepare 0.1M NaOH solution by dissolving 4 g of NaOH in 1 liter of water.
3. Hydrochloric acid.

Procedure

1. Dry the potassium hydrogen phthalate at 110 °C in oven for at least 1 hour. After the drying period remove the compound from the oven and allow it cool to room temperature in the desiccator.
2. Weigh between 0.7 and 0.9 g of the cooled potassium hydrogen phthalate into each of three, labeled, 250 mL Erlenmeyer flasks. Record the mass of the solid that is in each flask.
3. Add 30 mL of distilled or deionized water and two drops of phenolphthalein solution to each flask.
4. Fill the 50 mL burette with the sodium hydroxide solution.
5. Titrate the solution which is in each Erlenmeyer flask to the end point with the sodium hydroxide solution.
6. The end point color change is from colorless to light pink. Record the three endpoint volumes to the nearest 0.01 mL.
7. Take at least 35 mL of acetic acid solution.
8. Use a pipette to add 10 mL of the acetic acid solution to the 250 mL beaker.
9. Add about 140 mL of distilled or deionized water and a stirring bar to the beaker.
10. Place the beaker on a magnetic stirrer.
11. Use a clamp to suspend the electrodes in the solution.
12. The platinum electrodes must be completely submerged in the solution, but they should not interfere with operation of the stirring bar.
13. Adjust the stirring rate to yield a smoothly stirred solution.
14. Refill the burette with sodium hydroxide solution.
15. Measure the initial conductance of the stirred solution.

16. Add 1 mL portions of the sodium and the total volume of the added titrant solution after each addition.

17. Continue the titration until the end point has been passed by 100% i.e., until a total volume that is twice the end-point volume has been added.

18. Similarly dilute and titrate two, more 10 mL portions of the acetic acid solution.

19. After the titrations have been completed, store the electrodes in water.

Observation and Calculations

S. no.	Volume of NaOH	Conductance
1		
2		
3		
4		
5		
6		

1. Use the mass of potassium hydrogen phthalate (M.W. = 204.23) that was in each flask and the corresponding end point volume of the sodium hydroxide solution to calculate three values of the concentration (M) of the sodium hydroxide solution.

2. For each conductometric titration, plot conductance (y axis) as a function of the volume of the added sodium hydroxide solution. Draw a straight line through each of the two, linear portions in each titration curve. Determine the endpoint volume of each titration from the intersection of the two straight lines.

3. Use the endpoint volumes and the mean sodium hydroxide concentration to calculate three values of the concentration of the original acetic acid solution.

CHAPTER 11

Flame Photometry

Flame photometry is one of the branch of atomic spectroscopy in which the samples examined in the spectrometer are in the form of atoms. This is also known as flame atomic emission spectrometry. In this, the atoms under investigation are excited by light. Metallic salts (or metallic compounds) after dissolution in appropriate solvents when introduced into a flame (for instance: acetylene burning in oxygen at 3200 °C), turns into its vapors that essentially contain mostly atoms of the metal. Quite a few such gaseous metal atoms are usually raised to a particular high energy level that enables them to allow the emission of radiation characteristics features of the metal: for example – the characteristic flame colorations of metals frequently encountered in simple organic compounds such as : Na – yellow, Ca – brick-red ; Ba – apple-green. This forms the fundamental basis of **Flame Photometry.** The emission spectrum thus obtained is made up of a number of lines that actually originate from the resulting excited atoms or ions; and these steps may be shown diagrammatically as represented in Figure 11.1 below.

$$M^+A^- \ \rightleftharpoons \ M^+A^- \ \rightleftharpoons \ M^+A^-$$
$$\text{(Liquid)} \quad 1 \quad \text{(Vapour)} \quad \text{II} \quad \text{(Solid)}$$

$$\text{III}$$

$$M^\bullet_{(gas)} \ \xleftarrow{\ V\ } \ M_{(gas)} + A_{(gas)} \ \rightleftharpoons \ MA$$
$$\text{IV} \quad \text{(Gas)}$$

Fig. 11.1 Diagrammatic representation of emission spectrum from excited atoms or ions.

The various steps (I to V) in Figure above are explained as under:

(i)   The liquid sample containing a suitable compound of the metal ($M^+ A^-$) is aspirated into a flame, thereby converting it into its vapors or liquid droplets,

(ii) The evaporation of vapors (or droplets) give rise to the corresponding solid residue,

(iii) The vaporization of the solid residue into its gaseous state occurs,

(iv) The dissociation of the gaseous state into its constituent atoms, namely : M(gas) + A(gas) take place, that initially, is in ground state,

(v)   The thermal excitation of some atoms into their respective higher energy levels will lead ultimately to a condition whereby they radiate energy (flame emission) measured by Flame Emission Spectroscopy (FES).

Theory

The underlying principle of Flame Emission Spectroscopy (FES) may be explained when a liquid sample containing a metallic salt solution under investigation is introduced into a flame, the following steps normally take place in quick succession, namely:

(i)   The solvent gets evaporated leaving behind the corresponding solid salt,

(ii) The solid salt undergoes vaporization and gets converted into its respective gaseous state, and

(iii) The progressive dissociation of either a portion or all of the gaseous molecules gives rise to free neutral atoms or radicals.

The resulting neutral atoms are excited by the thermal energy of the flame which are fairly unstable, and hence instantly emit photons and eventually return to the ground state (*i.e.,* the lower energy state). The resulting emission spectrum caused by the emitted photons and its subsequent measurement forms the fundamental basis of FES.

Instrumentation

In general, Flame Photometers are designed and intended mainly for carrying out the assay of elements like: Sodium, Potassium, Calcium, and Lithium that possess the ability to give out an easily excited flame spectrum having sufficient intensity for rapid detection by a photocell.

Procedure

The compressed and filtered air (A) is first introduced into a Nebulizer (E) which creates a negative pressure (suction) enabling the liquid sample (C) to gain entry into the atomizer (E). Thus, it mixes with the stream of air as a fine droplet (mist) which goes into the burner (G). The fuel gas (D) introduced into the mixing chambers (F) at a given pressure gets in touch with the air and the mixture is ignited. Consequently, the radiation from the resulting flame (H) is made to pass through a convex lens (I) and ultimately through an optical filter (J) that allows specifically the radiation characteristic of the element under examination to pass through the photocell (K). Finally, the output from the photocell is adequately amplified (L) and subsequently measured on an appropriate sensitive digital-read-out device (Figure 11.2).

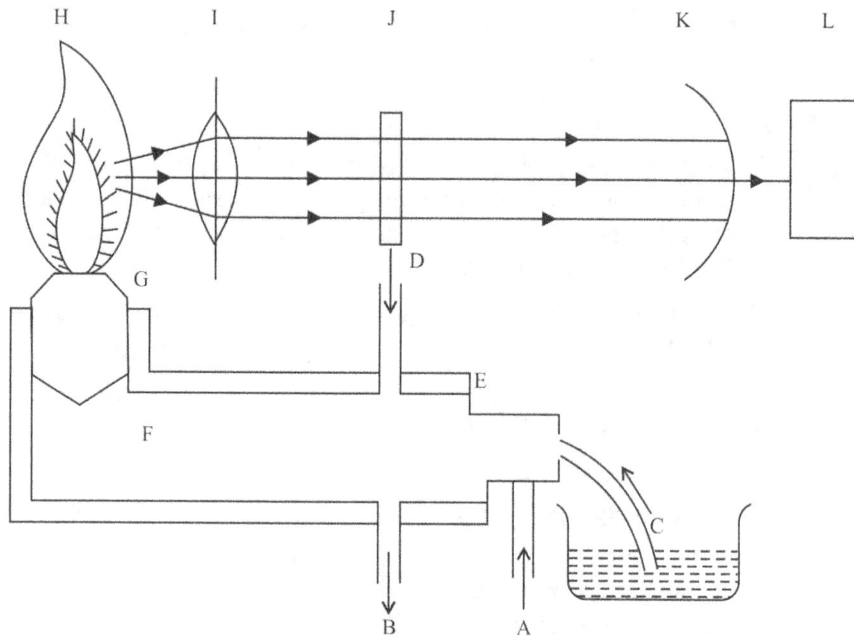

Fig. 11.2 Lay out of a flame photometer

A = Inlet for compressed Air,

B = Drain outlet (to maintain constant pressure head in the mixing Chamber),

C = Liquid sample (sucked into the Nebulizer),

D = Inlet for Fuel-Gas to the Laminar-Flow-Burner,

E = Nebulizer to atomize the liquid sample,

F = Mixing Chamber for Fuel Gas, Compressed Air, and Atomize Liquid Sample,

G = Burner,

H = Flame,

I = Convex lens,

J = Optical filter to transmit only a strong-line of the element,

K = photo cell

L = Amplifier to amplify the feeble electrical impulse and a built-in direct read-out device.

Experiment 11.1

Determination of Sodium and Potassium Ion Concentrations in Solution

Theory

Flame photometry is a relatively old instrumental analysis method. As an analytical method, atomic emission is a fast, simple, and sensitive method for the determination of trace metal ions in solution. Because of the very narrow (0.01 nm) and characteristic emission lines from the gas-phase atoms in the flame plasma, the method is relatively free of interferences from other elements.

The method is suitable for many metallic elements, especially for those metals that are easily excited to higher energy levels at the relatively cool temperatures of some flames - Li, Na, K, Rb, Cs, Ca, Cu, Sr, and Ba. Metalloids and nonmetals generally do not produce isolated neutral atoms in a flame, but mostly as polyatomic radicals and ions. Therefore, nonmetallic elements are not suitable for determination by flame emission spectroscopy, except for very few and under very specialized conditions.

Chemicals required

1. **Standard sodium stock solution, 100.0 ppm**

    (i) Accurately weigh out by difference 0.1271 g of reagent grade NaCl into a small weighing bottle. It is very difficult and time consuming to weigh out exactly this amount. Get it as close as you reasonably can, record the exact mass, and correct your concentrations accordingly.

    Note: Mol. Weight of NaCl = 58.5

    58.5 g NaCl/litre = 1000 ppm of NaCl

    58.5/23 g NaCl/litre = 1000 ppm for Na

    0.1271 of NaCl/500 mL = 100 ppm of Na

(ii) Carefully transfer the salt quantitatively into a 500 mL volumetric flask. Use a few squirts of deionized water from wash bottle on the weighing bottle and the sides of the flask to wash all of it down into the flask.

(iii) Add about 100 mL of deionized water to the flask, swirl several times, and dissolve all of the salt before diluting to volume with deionized water.

2. Standard potassium stock solution, 100.0 ppm

Similarly make the stock solution for potassium (atomic weight of K = 39 and Cl = 33.5).

3. Unknown solution

Obtain the unknown sample and carefully dilute to 100 mL mark with deionized water.

Procedure

1. Preparation of standard calibration solution

(i) Pipette out 10.00, 20.00, 30.00, 40.00, 50.00, 60.0, 70.0, 80.0, 90.0 mL of the standard 100 ppm sodium solution into different volumetric flasks.

(ii) This will give the concentration range of 10 to 90 ppm respectively. Dilute carefully to the mark with deionized water and mix thoroughly.

2. Instructions for use of the Flame Photometer

(i) Ensure that the photometer drain is leading into a sink and that the instrument is connected to gas, air and electricity supplies. Ensure the main supply gas tap is off.

(ii) Turn the sensitivity and instrument gas controls fully counter clockwise.

(iii) Insert the sodium optical filter (589 nm).

(iv) Switch on the instrument and unclamp the galvanometer by turning counter clockwise.

(v) Open the mica window, turn on the mains gas supply, light the gas and close the window.

(vi) Turn on the air supply control and adjust the sir pressure to 10 lb/in^2. Leave for 1-2 minutes to stabilize.

(vii)   Place a beaker of distilled water into position at the left hand side of the instrument and insert the narrow draw tube into it to allow water to pass thorugh the photometer.

(viii) Once set up, the photometer must have water running through it at all times when a salt solution is not being measured. The rate of uptake is fast, so make sure there is always enough water in the beaker.

(ix)   Adjust the gas control to give a flame with a large central blue cone then, with water passing through the instrument, slowly close the gas control until ten separate blue cones just form.

(x)   Set the galvanometer to zero using the set zero control.

(xi)   Replace the distilled water with the NaCl solution (100 ppm standard) and adjust the sensitivity control till the galvanometer reads 100.

(xii)   Quickly but carefully, replace the NaCl standard with standards of decreasing concentration.

(xiii) Run water through the instrument again for 1-2 min then place the draw tube into a beaker containing the unknown sachet solution and note the galvanometer reading.

(xiv)   Run water through the instrument again and replace the sodium with the potassium filter (766 nm).

(xv)   Repeat the above procedure with the KCl standards, setting to 100 with most concentrated KCl standard, then reading the others in reverse order. Then, read the unknown solution.

(xvi)   Finally, run water through the instrument until the flame appears free of color again.

(xvii) When the instrument is no longer required, switch off in the following sequence:

    (a)   Turn off the gas control and the mains gas supply

    (b)   Wait for the flame to die out.

    (c)   Turn off the air supply.

    (d)   Switch off the electricity.

    (e)   Clamp the galvanometer.

Observation and Calculation

Make a calibration curve by plotting the emission intensities as a function of sodium and potassium concentration separately. Determine the concentration of sodium and potassium unknown sample from the calibration curve. Multiply with the dilution factor to get the concentration in original solution.

CHAPTER 12

Polarimetry

The classical electromagnetic theory of light put forward by Maxwell advocates that the electric and magnetic fields associated with a beam of monochromatic light vibrate in all directions perpendicular to the direction of propagation of light. In fact, there exists an indefinite number of planes that pass through the line of propagation, and an ordinary light usually vibrates in all the planes. This is also referred to as **unpolarized light**. Under certain specific circumstances, the vibrations may all be restricted to one direction only, in the perpendicular plane and this is termed as **plane-polarized light (Fig. 12.1)**.

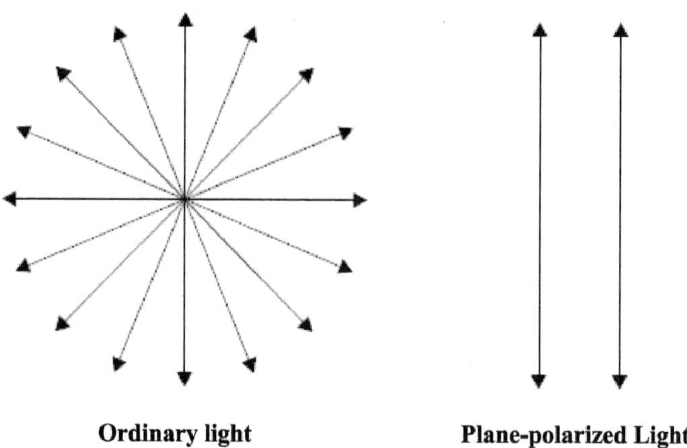

Fig. 12.1

A few crystalline substances, for instance : Iceland spar, Calcite (a form of $CaCO_3$) or Polaroid, possess different refractive indices for light whose field oscillates either perpendicular or parallel to the principal plane of the crystal. Thus, an ordinary light (unpolarized light) gets converted into a plane-polarized light by simply passing it through a lens made of the above cited materials and traditionally called a **Nicol prism** (after **William Nicol - the inventor**). Therefore, an optically active substance is one that rotates the plane of polarized light. In other words, certain specific substances by virtue of their internal structure may be able to transmit only such vibrations that are oriented along certain directions and entirely block vibrations in other directions. The rotation of the plane of polarized light and hence the optical activity may be detected and measured accurately by an instrument known as the polarimeter (Fig. 12.2).

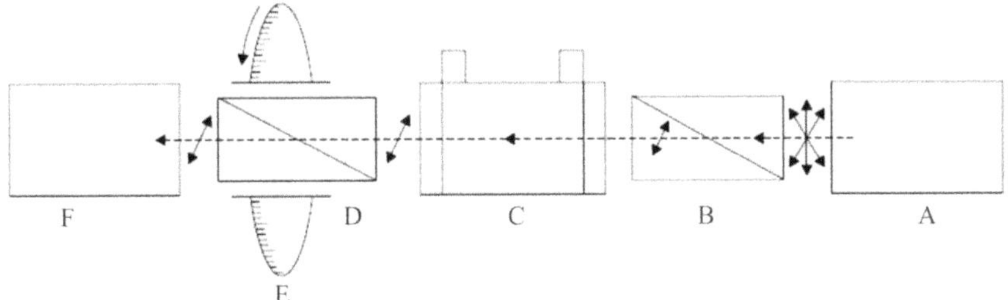

A = Collimated monochromatic light source,

B = Polarizing prism (Nicol),

C = Polarimeter glass tube (20 cm) with glass windows,

D = Analyzing rotator prism (Nicol),

E = Circular scale with vernier,

F = Null detector (Eye or Photoelectric Cell).

Fig. 12.2 Optical system of a polarimeter.

The underlying principle of a polarimeter is that light from the source; usually a sodium vapour lamp, first gets collimated at A, and subsequently falls upon polarizer B (a **calcite prism**). The polarizer permits only the light polarized in a particular direction to pass it. The emergent polarized ray now passes through the sample under investigation, kept in the polarimeter glass tube C to the analyzer D, which happens to be another polarizing prism. The analyzing rotator prism D (**Nicol**) is fixed in such a manner that it can be rotated easily about the axis of the incident light ray. Two situations arise when the analyzing rotator prism (D) is put into action, *firstly*, the prism being parallel to the plane of polarization of the incident light – the net result is that the intensity of light reaching the Null detector F is maximum; and *secondly*, the prism being perpendicular to the plane of the polarized light – the net result is observed by the intensity of light reaching the detector as minimum. Hence, the overall difference in the position of the analyzer, as noted from the circular scale E, that provides minimum light intensity with and without the sample in the cell is the observed 'rotation' of the sample in question.

Experiment 12.1

To Determine Sugar by Polarimetric Method

Theory

Polarimetry is a non-destructive technique for measuring the optical activity of several organic and inorganic compounds. Optically active compounds like sugar rotate the plane polarized light when passed through it. Degree of rotation depends on the structure of the molecule and the concentration of the compound. Specific rotation of each substance is calculated by the formula:

$$[\alpha]_D^T = \frac{[\alpha]\text{abs}}{1 \times c}$$

where,

$[\alpha]_D^T$ is the specific rotation of the compound at temperature T using D line of the sodium spectrum as the source of light.

$[\alpha]$ abs is the observed angle of rotation

l is the path length in decimeter

c is the concentration of the compound in g/100 mL

Chemicals required

1. Dextrose

2. Water

Procedure

1. Prepare 5, 10 and 15 % solution of dextrose.

2. Measure the angle of rotation for these solutions and record as in Table 12.1.

3. Similarly measure the angle of rotate on for the unknown sample.

Observation and Calculations

Table 12.1 Measurements of specific rotation

S. No.	% solution	Angle of rotation
1.	Distilled water	
2.	5 % dextrose solution	
3.	10 % dextrose solution	
4.	15 % dextrose solution	
5.	Unknown sample	

Calculate Specific rotation of each substance by the formula:

$$[\alpha]_D^T = \frac{[\alpha]\text{abs}}{1 \times c}$$

Plot a graph between specific rotation and concentration of the dextrose solutions. Read out the concentration of the unknown sample from the graph.

Experiment 12.2

To Determine Levodopa by Polarimetric Method

Theory

The optical rotation of a number of pure pharmaceutical substances like Levodopa may be measured accurately by noting the angle through which the plane of polarization is rotated when polarized light passes through the substance, i.e., liquid or solid. It has been observed that the specific rotation of levodopa in the visible region is rather on the lower side i.e., $[\alpha]_D^{20} = -12°$ in 1M hydrochloric acid). Therefore, it is necessary to enhance the optical rotation to a reasonable extent by some suitable means. It is, however, achieved by the formation of a complex with hexamine.

Chemicals required

1. 0.2 g Dried levodopa

2. 5.0 g Hexamine

3. 1M Hydrochloric acid

Procedure

1. Dissolve a quantity equivalent to 0.2 *g* of the dried substance and 5 *g* of hexamine in 10 mL of 1M hydrochloric acid, add sufficient 1M HCl to produce 25 mL.

2. Allow to stand for 3 hours protected from light.

3. The optical rotation is measured by a previously calibrated polarimeter.

Observation and Calculations

Calculate Specific rotation of Levodopa by the formula:

$$[\alpha]_D^T = \frac{[\alpha]\text{abs}}{1 \times c}$$

CHAPTER 13

Ion Exchange Chromatography

Introduction

Ion exchange chromatography is a separation technique used for purification or analysis of molecules based their charge. The method can be used to separate charged molecules from uncharged ones or it can separate molecules of different charge from one another. Ion exchange is probably the most frequently used chromatographic technique for the separation and purification of proteins, polypeptides, nucleic acids, polynucleotides, and other charged biomolecules. The reasons for the success of ion exchange are its widespread applicability, high resolving power, high capacity, and the simplicity and controllability of the method.

Principle of the Method

Ionizable chemical groups are immobilized on a solid support such as cellulose or agarose. The support, or resin, is usually maintained in a column. Molecules of opposite charge can bind the column by electrostatic interaction while uncharged residues will pass through. Once bound to the column, molecules can be released with salt (NaCl is commonly used, but other salts can be used also). The salt ions compete for interaction for the column, and the molecule of interest is released. Hence the term "ion exchange".

Molecules having different charges can be separated from one another by gradually increasing the salt concentration. This is achieved with a gradient of increasing salt concentration in the solution being passed through the column. Lower charged groups are released at low salt concentrations because they are weakly bound. Highly charged molecules are more tightly bound and require higher salt concentration to release them. Thus molecules are released from the column according to the magnitude of their charge.

It should be noted that pH of the column buffers can have a profound effect on ion exchange chromatography. Both the ion exchange resin and the molecule binding to it are charged molecules with a defined pKa. If the pH is on one side of the pKa, the molecule will be uncharged, and it will be charged on the other. Also, the difference between the pH and the pKa will determine how much of the resin is ionized that in turn will determine how tightly other molecules will bind.

The charged resin can be of two types: cation exchangers and anion exchangers. The name of the resin refers to the molecules being exchanged, not the molecule bound to the resin. Cation exchangers bind positively charged molecules and anion exchangers (Figure 13.1) bind negative ones.

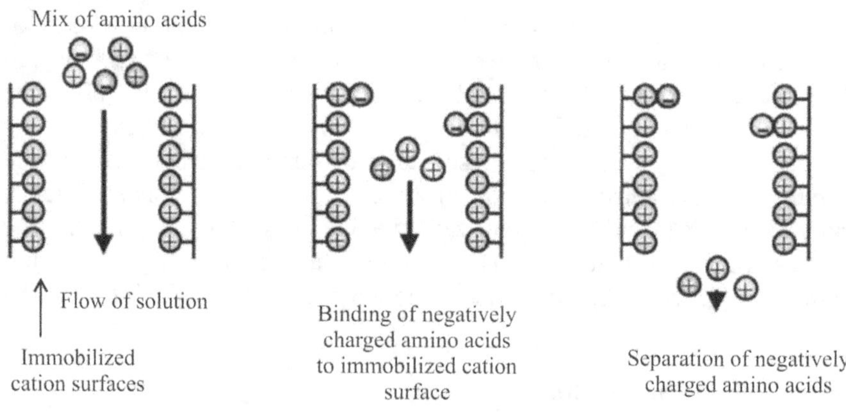

Fig. 13.1 Anion exchanger.

The matrix of ion-exchanger

An ion exchanger consists of an insoluble matrix to which charged groups have been covalently bound. The charged groups are associated with mobile counter-ions. These counter-ions can be reversibly exchanged with other ions of the same charge without altering the matrix. The matrix may be based on inorganic compounds, synthetic resins or polysaccharides. The characteristics of the matrix determine its chromatographic properties such as efficiency, capacity and recovery as well as its chemical stability, mechanical strength and flow properties. The nature of the matrix will also affect its behavior towards biological substances and the maintenance of biological activity.

Capacity of ion-exchanger

The capacity of an ion-exchanger is a quantitative measure of its ability to take up exchangeable counter-ions and is therefore of major importance. The capacity may be expressed as total ionic capacity, available capacity or dynamic capacity. The total ionic capacity is the number of charged substituent groups per gram dry ion-exchanger or per mL swollen gel. Total capacity can be measured by titration with a strong acid or base.

The actual amount of protein which can be bound to an ion-exchanger, under defined experimental conditions, is referred to as the available capacity for the gel. If the defined conditions include the flow rate at which the gel was operated, the amount bound is referred to as the dynamic capacity for the ion-exchanger. Available and dynamic capacities depend upon:

The properties of the protein: The properties of the protein which determine the available or dynamic capacity on a particular ion exchange matrix are its molecular size and its charge/pH relationship. The capacity of an ion-exchanger is thus different for different proteins.

The properties of the ion-exchanger: Properties of the ion exchange matrix which determine its available capacity for a particular protein are the exclusion limit of the matrix, and the type and number of the charged substituents. High available capacity is obtained by having a matrix which is macro-porous and highly substituted with ionic groups which maintain their charge over a wide range of experimental conditions. Non-porous matrices have considerably lower capacity than porous matrices, but higher efficiency due to shorter diffusion distances.

Experimental conditions: The experimental conditions which affect the observed capacity are pH, the ionic strength of the buffer, the nature of the counter-ion, the flow rate and the temperature. The flow rate is of particular importance with respect to dynamic capacity, which decreases as the flow rate is increased. These conditions should always be taken into consideration when comparing available capacities for different ion exchangers.

Experiment 13.1

To Determine Ion-Exchange Capacity of Resins

Chemicals required

1. Ion-exchange resin granules
2. Hydrochloric acid
3. Sodium hydroxide
4. Phenolphthalein
5. Methyl orange

Procedure

1. Preparation of cation exchange resin

(i) Measure 30 mL of Ion Exchange Resin (granule), transfer into a glass tube for chromatography (about 3 cm in internal diameter), flow 1,000 mL of diluted hydrochloric acid at a rate of 15-20 mL per minute, and wash by flowing water at the same rate.

(ii) Measure 10 mL of the washings, and perform the test for Chloride. Wash with water until the amount is not more than the amount equivalent to 0.3 mL of 0.01M hydrochloric acid.

2. Preparation of Anion exchange resin

(i) Measure 30 mL of Ion Exchange Resin (granule), transfer into a glass tube for chromatography (about 3 cm in internal diameter), flow 1,000 mL of sodium hydroxide solution (1-25) at a rate of 15-20 mL per minute, and wash by flowing water at the same rate.

(ii) Wash with water until the washings become neutral with phenolphthalein TS.

3. Determination of total solid

(i) Solids not less than 25%.

(ii) Weigh 10.0 g of sample A. In case of cation exchange resin, dry at 100 °C for 12 hours, and weigh again; in case of anion exchange resin, dry at 40 °C for 12 hours in a vacuum desiccator at 4 kPa, and weigh again.

4. Total ion exchange capacity of cation exchange resin

(i) Weigh accurately about 5 g of prepared sample.

(ii) Add 500 mL of 0.2M sodium hydroxide, measured accurately and allow to stand for 12 hours while shaking occasionally.

(iii) Measure exactly 10 mL of the supernatant, and titrate with 0.05M sulfuric acid (indicator: 3 drops of methyl orange TS).

(iv) Perform a blank test in the same manner.

5. Total ion exchange capacity of anion exchange resin

(i) Weigh accurately about 5 g of sample a prepared for the Purity Tests.

(ii) Add 500 mL of 0.2 mol/L hydrochloric acid, exactly measured, and allow to stand for 12 hours while shaking occasionally.

(iii) Measure exactly 10 mL of the supernatant, and titrate with 0.1 mol/L sodium hydroxide (indicator: 3 drops of phenolphthalein TS).

(iv) Perform a blank test in the same manner.

Observation and Calculations

1. To calculate the total ion exchange capacity of cation exchange resin

Total ion exchange capacity =

$$\frac{\begin{array}{c}\text{Volume of 0.05M } H_2SO_4 \\ \text{consumed in blank test}\end{array} \times \begin{array}{c}\text{Volume of 0.05M } H_2SO_4 \\ \text{consumed in this test}\end{array}}{\text{Weight of sample (g)} \times \text{Solide}(\%)} \times 100$$

$$= \text{........milliequivalents/g}$$

2. **To calculate the total ion exchange capacity of anion exchange resin**

Total ion exchange capacity =

$$\dfrac{\text{Volume of 0.1M NaOH consumed in blank test} \times \text{Volume of 0.1M NaOH consumed in this test}}{\text{Weight of sample (g)} \times \text{Solide}(\%)} \times 100$$

= ……..milliequivalents/g

CHAPTER 14

Electrophoresis

Principles of Electrophoresis

Electrophoresis is the process of moving charged molecules in solution by applying an electric field across the mixture (Figure 14.1). Because molecules in an electric field move with a speed dependent on their charge, shape, and size, electrophoresis has been extensively used for molecular separations. As an analytical tool, electrophoresis is simple and relatively rapid. It is used mainly for analysis and purification of very large molecules such as proteins and nucleic acids, but can also be applied to simpler charged molecules, including charged sugars, amino acids, peptides, nucleotides, and simple ions.

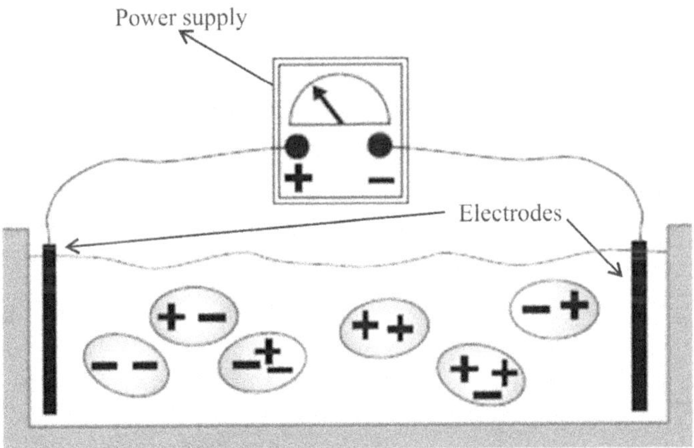

Fig. 14.1 Basic arrangement for electrophoresis.

Electrophoresis of macromolecules is normally carried out by applying a thin layer of a sample to a solution stabilized by a porous matrix. Under the influence of an applied voltage, different species of molecules in the sample move through the matrix at different velocities. At the end of the separation, the different species are detected as bands at

187

different positions in the matrix. A matrix is required because the electric current passing through the electrophoresis solution generates heat, which causes diffusion and convective mixing of the bands in the absence of a stabilizing medium. The matrix is composed of a number of different materials, including paper, cellulose acetate, or gels made of polyacrylamide, agarose, or starch.

Gels can be of all sizes, depending on the separation distance required and the amount of sample. Analytical tube gels are commonly cast in glass tubes with an inside diameter of 1-5 mm and a length of 5-25 cm. Preparative tube gels may range up to 10 cm in diameter to accommodate larger amounts of material. At the other extreme, gels run in capillaries 50-100 μm in diameter and 30-100 cm long provide very high resolution and rapid separations of very small amounts of sample. Vertical slab gels are normally cast between a pair of glass plates for support. A chamber is constructed by separating the two plates with spacer strips down the edges of the plates, then sealing the edges and bottom to form a liquid tight box or "sandwich". Slab gels range in size from 2.5 cm square (between microscope cover slips) to 30-150 cm square and from <0.05 mm to >5 mm thick.

Experiment 14.1

Demonstration of Separation of Proteins by SDS Gel Electrophoresis

Theory

In SDS polyacrylamide gel electrophoresis (SDS-PAGE) separations, migration is determined not by intrinsic electric charge of polypeptides but by molecular weight. Sodium dodecylsulphate (SDS) is an anionic detergent that denatures proteins by wrapping the hydrophobic tail around the polypeptide backbone. For almost all proteins, SDS binds at a ratio of approximately 1.4 g SDS per gram of protein, thus conferring a net negative charge to the polypeptide in proportion to its length. The SDS also disrupts hydrogen bonds, blocks hydrophobic interactions, and substantially unfolds the protein molecules, minimizing differences in molecular form by eliminating the tertiary and secondary structures. The SDS - denatured and reduced polypeptides are flexible rods with uniform negative charge per unit length. Thus, because molecular weight is essentially a linear function of peptide chain length, in sieving gels the proteins separate by molecular weight.

Chemicals required

1. **Acrylamide solution:** Dissolve 60 g of Acrylamide and 1.6 g bisacrylamide in doubly distilled water and make up the volume up to 200 mL.

   Note: Store up to 3 months at 4 °C in the dark.

2. **4×Resolving gel buffer:** Dissolve 36.3 g of Tris in about 150 mL of doubly distilled water. Adjust the pH of the solution to 8.8 using HCl. Make the volume of the solution up to 200 mL with doubly distilled water if necessary.

   Note: Store up to 3 months at 4 °C.

3. **4 × Stacking gel buffer:** Dissolve 3.0 g of Tris in about 40 mL of doubly distilled water. Adjust the pH of the solution to 6.8 using

HCl. Make the volume of the solution up to 50 mL with doubly distilled water if necessary.

Note: Store up to 3 months at 4 °C.

4. **10% SDS:** Dissolve 10.0 g of SDS in 100 mL of doubly distilled water.

    Note: Store up to 6 months at room temperature.

5. **10% Ammonium persulphate (initiator):** Dissolve 0.1 g of Ammonium persulphate in 1 mL of doubly distilled water.

    Note: Store up to 6 months at room temperature.

6. **Resolving gel overlay:** Dissolve 25 mL of 4 × Resolving gel buffer in 1.0 mL of 10% SDS and make up the volume up to 100 mL with doubly distilled water.

7. **2×Treatment buffer:** Mix 4 × stacking gel buffer, 2.5 mL; 10% SDS 4.0 mL; Glycerol 2.0 mL; Bromophenol blue 2.0 mg; Dithiothreitol, 0.31 g and make the volume up to 100.0 mL with doubly distilled water.

    Note: Store in 0.5 ml aliquots at –20 °C for up to 6 months.

8. **Tank buffer:** Dissolve Tris; 30.28 g; Glycine 144.13 g; SDS 10 g in sufficient doubly distilled water and then make up the volume up to 10 liter.

9. **Water-saturated n-butanol:** Mix 50 mL n-butanol in 5 mL of water.

Procedure

1. **Prepare the separating gel**

    (i)   Assemble the vertical slab gel unit in the dual-gel casting stand. Use 1.5 mm or 0.75 mm spacers.

    (ii) In a 125 mL side-arm vacuum flask, mix either 40 mL (0.75 mm) or 80 mL (1.5 mm) of resolving gel solution, leaving out the ammonium persulphate and the resolving gel solution.

    (iii) Stopper the flask and apply a water vacuum for several minutes to deaerate the solution while swirling the flask.

    (iv) Add the resolving gel solution and ammonium persulphate and gently swirl the flask to mix, being careful not to generate bubbles.

(v)   Pipette the solution down the spacer into each sandwich to a level about 4 cm from the top. A 25 mL pipette works well for this step.

(vi)   Fill a transfer pipette or syringe with water-saturated n-butanol (or water or resolving gel overlay). Position the pipette or needle at about a 45° angle with the point at the top of the acrylamide next to a spacer. Gently apply approximately 0.3 mL of n-butanol. Repeat on the other side of the slab next to the other spacer. The n-butanol will layer evenly across the entire surface after a minute or two. Repeat this process to overlay the second slab. A very sharp liquid-gel interface will be visible when the gel has polymerized. This should be visible within 10-20 min. The gel should be fully polymerized in about 1 hr.

(vii)   After polymerization, tilt the casting stand to pour off the overlay and rinse the surfaces of the gels twice with resolving gel overlay. Gels may be stored at this point. The stacking gel is cast later. Remove the n-butanol and add approximately 10 ml of 1 × resolving gel overlay solution to the top of each sandwich, seal with plastic wrap, and store flat at 4 °C. Or store gels submerged flat in 1 × resolving gel overlay at 4 °C for up to 1 week.

(viii) Add approximately 1 mL of resolving gel overlay to each gel and allow the gels to sit while preparing the stacking gel.

2. Prepare the stacking gel

(i)   In a 50 mL side-arm vacuum flask, mix 10 mL (for 0.75-mm-thick gels) or 20 mL (for 1.5-mm-thick gels) of stacking gel solution, leaving out the ammonium persulphate and the stacking gel solution.

(ii)   Deaerate as in step (iii) above.

(iii)   Add the ammonium persulphate and stacking gel solution. Gently swirl the flask to mix.

(iv)   Pour off resolving gel overlay from the gel. Remove all liquid before proceeding.

(v)   Fill each sandwich with stacking gel solution and insert a comb into each sandwich, taking care not to trap any bubbles below the teeth of the comb. Oxygen will inhibit polymerization, and bubbles will cause a local distortion in the gel surface at the bottom of the wells.

(vi)   Allow the gel to sit for at least 30 min. A very sharp interface will be visible when the gel has polymerized. This should be visible within 10-20 min. The gel should be fully polymerized after 1 hr. In general, stacking gels should be cast just before use. The complete gel can be stored overnight at 4 °C, however, with little effect on resolution, if covered and the comb left in place.

3. Prepare the sample

(i)   Combine equal volumes of protein sample and 2 × treatment buffers in a tube and place the tube in a boiling-water bath for 90 s. If using dry samples, add equal volumes of water and 2 × treatment buffer and heat in a boiling-water bath for 90 s. If the gels will be stained with Coomassie Blue, use a starting sample protein concentration of 10-20 mg/mL (i.e., 10-20 µg/µL). This will be diluted by the 2 × treatment buffer to give 5–10 µg/µL. For complex mixtures (e.g., cell lysates), 50 µg of protein (5–10 µL of treated sample) per lane is recommended. For highly purified proteins, 0.5-5 µg per lane is usually adequate. Silver staining requires 10- to 100-fold less protein per lane.

(ii)   Place samples briefly on ice until ready for use. The treated sample can be stored at 20 °C for 6 months for future runs.

Note: The SDS may precipitate if tubes are left on ice for long periods of time.

4. Load the gels

(i)   Slowly remove the combs from the gels, raising the comb up to avoid disturbing the well dividers.

(ii)   Rinse each well with tank buffer, invert the casting stand to drain the wells, and return the stand to an upright position.

(iii)   Fill each well with tank buffer.

(iv)   Using a pipette with a long, thin tip, gently load 5-10 µL of sample beneath the buffer in each well. Load every well with the same volume of sample. If the well is not needed, load with 1 × sample buffer containing standard protein or no sample.

(v)   If protein molecular weight standards are used, load one or two wells with 5-10 µL of the standard mixture. If the gel is to be stained with Coomassie Blue, this volume should contain 0.2-1 µg of each standard component. If the gel is to be silver stained, use 10-50 ng of each component.

5. Run the gel

(i)   Fill the lower buffer chamber with 4 l of tank buffer. Install the sealing gaskets on the upper buffer chamber and put it in place on the gel sandwiches. Remove the lower cams and cam the sandwiches to the bottom of the upper buffer chamber. Put the upper buffer chamber in place on the heat exchanger in the lower buffer chamber.

(ii)   Adjust the height of the tank buffer in the lower buffer chamber until the sandwiches are fully immersed in buffer. If bubbles are trapped under the end of the sandwiches, coax them away with a pipette.

(iii) Add a spin bar to the lower buffer chamber and center the chamber on a magnetic stirrer. When the lower buffer is stirred, the temperature of the buffer remains uniform. This is important because uneven heating distorts the band pattern of the gel and leads to smiling.

(iv)   Carefully fill the upper buffer chamber with tank buffer. Do not pour buffer into the sample wells, because it will wash the sample out.

(v)   Put the lid on the gel unit and connect it to the Power Supply. The cathode is connected to the upper buffer chamber.

(vi)   Turn on the power supply and adjust the voltage to 300.

(vii) Adjust the current to 30 mA per 1.5-mm-thick gel and 15 mA per 0.75-mm-thick gel. Start the electrophoresis. The voltage should start at about 70-80 V, but will increase during the run. Keep a record of the voltage and current readings so that future runs can be compared and current leaks or incorrectly made buffers can be detected.

(viii) When the tracking dye reaches the bottom of the gel, turn the power supply off and disconnect the power cables.

6. Disassemble the gel sandwiches

(i) Remove the buffer and disassemble the sandwiches by gently loosening and sliding away both spacers. Slip an extra spacer or a Hoefer Wonder Wedge into the bottom edge and separate the plates. Carefully lift the gel into a tray of staining solution.

Experiment 14.2

Separation of DNA by Gel Electrophoresis

Theory

Since nucleic acids are negatively charged, DNA will migrate through the gel in the direction toward the positive pole of the electric field. Since the gel acts as a sieve, it normally impedes the movement of larger molecules. Therefore, smaller molecules will migrate faster along the gel toward the positive electrode (anode). The rate at which these molecules travel are inversely proportional to their molecular weight. The electrophoretic mobility of DNA through agarose gel is dependent on the molecular size of DNA. For example Linear DNA travels through the agarose gel matrix at rate inversely proportional to $\log_{10}$ of its molecular weight. In order to determine accurately the molecular weights of the unknown fragments, all samples that are being analyzed using gel electrophoresis will usually be run in parallel with known standards or DNA ladders (i.e., DNA fragments of known molecular weights).

Material required

1. Agarose powder or pre-cast agarose gels

2. Loading dye (e.g., bromophenol blue)

3. TAE or TBE Electrophoresis Buffer (20X stock and 1X stock)

4. Gel electrophoresis separation trays or chambers with safety lid, solid platinum wire and electrodes

5. Gel casting tray or holder (Plexiglas) with end dams and well-combs.

6. Power supply (e.g., batteries - 9 volts or a variable power supply with the ability to run 3 chambers simultaneously)

7. 10 μL micropipette with disposable tips

8. DNA to be separated (usually genarated from spooling)

9. DNA ladders or "standards"

10. Marker dyes (for the DNA simulation experiment) e.g., bromo-phenol blue, janus green, Orange G, Safranin O, Xylene Cyanol.

Procedure

1. The hot agarose solution is usually poured into a Plexiglas holder (tray) and is allowed to solidify onto that support for 10-15 min. During the cooling process, the hot agarose solution becomes polymerized into a semi-solid matrix or gel.

2. This chamber is now filled with buffer to cover the gel to a depth of usually about 1-2 cm in depth. This important step is to ensure that the electric current should flow from the positive pole to the negative pole at opposite ends of the gel, thus promoting separation of the macromolecule sample.

3. A well comb is used to imprint a series of small wells at one end of the gel. The well comb is inserted before the gel is poured. The wells function as reservoirs for holding the DNA sample.

4. The DNA ladders or "standards" should be loaded into wells either on the right or left of the slab of gel so that the macromolecules in the "test" well can be easily compared.

5. The samples of DNA fragments to be electrophoresed, can be mixed with a loading buffer containing a tracking dye usually bromophenol blue, that will enable us to track the samples as they migrate from each well.

6. Loading the wells with the mixture of macromolecules should be carried out using a micropipette to ensure that a constant volume of test mixture is loaded into each well. It is important to change the tip of the micropipette after loading each standard to prevent contamination of the test sample.

7. An electric field used in gel electrophoresis is normally provided by a variable power supply.

8. The anode (positive) connected to the electrophoresis chamber will usually be colored red and the cathode (negative) black.

9. The electric current is usually turned off after a run time of 10-40 minutes depending on the amount of sample mixture. For example, a 5 μL of sample may require a run time of about 40 minutes using a voltage of nine volts, whereas a 15 μL sample may require a run time of approximately 1.25 hours.

10. The DNA fragments should be separated since they migrate according to their molecular size.

11. Once the loading dye has reached the top of the gel, the electrophoresis procedure is deemed complete.

12. Now gel is stained with Methylene blue that can bind loosely with the phosphate backbone of DNA to some degree, thus producing visible bands on the gels.

13. If the gel is allowed to stain for five minutes, the bands of separated DNA are usually quite prominent.

14. The final step would include plating the gel in a tray of water and allowing it to "destain" for approximately 60 minutes.

15. The gel is then removed from the tray and can be viewed immediately using a UV light box. This is done since methylene blue stains fade rapidly after it is used.

CHAPTER 15

Thin-layer Chromatography

Thin-layer chromatography (TLC) is a very important technique for the rapid separation and qualitative analysis of small amounts of material. The technique is closely related to column chromatography. In fact, TLC can be considered simply column chromatography in reverse, with the solvent ascending the adsorbent rather than descending. Because of close relationship and similar principles, column chromatography should be read before the thin layer chromatography.

Principles of Thin-layer Chromatography

Like column chromatography, thin-layer chromatography is a solid-liquid partitioning technique. However, the moving, liquid phase is not allowed to percolate down the adsorbent; it ascend a thin layer of adsorbent coated onto a backing support. The most typical backing is a glass plate, but other materials are also used. A thin layer of adsorbent is spread onto the plate and allowed to dry. A coated and dried plate of glass is called a thin-layer plate, or thin-layer slide (the reference to slide comes about because microscope slide are often used to prepare small thin-layer plates). When a thin layer plate is placed upright in a vessel that contains a shallow layer of solvent the solvent ascends the layer of adsorbent on the plate by capillary action.

In thin-layer chromatography, the sample is applied to the plate before the solvent is allowed to ascend the adsorbent layer. The sample is usually applied as a small spot near the base of the plate, and this technique is often referred to as spotting. The plate is spotted by repeated applications of a sample solution from a small capillary pipette. When the filled pipette touches the plate, capillary action delivers its contents to the plate, and a small spot is formed.

As the solvent ascends the plate, the sample is partitioned between the moving, liquid phase and the stationary, solid phase. During this process, one is said to be developing, or running, the thin layer plate. In development, the various components in the applied mixture are separated. The separation is based on the many equilibrations the solutes experience between the moving and stationary phases (Figure 15.1).

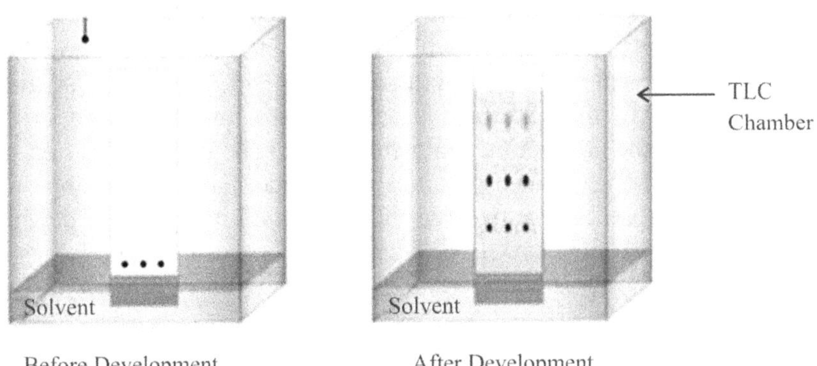

Fig. 15.1

A separation results from the differences in the rates at which the individual components of the mixture advance upwards on the plate. When many substances are present in a mixture, each has its own characteristic solubility and absorptivity properties, depending on the functional groups present in its structure. In general, the stationary phase is strongly polar and strongly binds polar substances. The moving liquid phase is usually less polar or even non-polar. Thus, while substances that are the most polar travel slowly upwards, or not all non-polar substances travel more rapidly if the solvent is sufficiently non-polar.

Preparation of thin-layer slides and plates

The two adsorbent materials most often used for TLC are alumina G (aluminum oxide) and silica gel G (silicic acid). The adsorbent materials are otherwise like those used in column chromatography; the adsorbents used in column chromatography have a larger particle size, however. The material for thin-layer work is a fine powder.

Microscopic slide TLC plates

For qualitative work such as identification the number of components in a mixture or trying to establish that two compounds are identical, small TLC plates made from microscope slides is especially convenient. Although numerous solvents can be used to prepare slurry, methylene chloride is probably the most convenient solvent. It has the two advantages of low boiling point (40 °C) and inability to cause the adsorbent to set or form lumps. The low boiling point means that it is not necessary to dry the coated slides in an oven.

Preparation of slurry

The slurry is most conveniently prepared in a 4-oz wide-mouthed screw-cap jar. About 3 mL of methylene chloride is required for each gram of silica gel G for smooth slurry without lumps, the silica gel should be added to the solvent while the mixture is being either stirred or swirled. Adding solvent to the adsorbent usually causes lumps to form in the mixture. When the addition is complete, the cap should be placed on the jar tightly and the jar shaken vigorously to ensure thorough mixing. The slurry may be stored, in the tightly capped jar, until it is to be used. More methylene chloride may have to be added to replace evaporation losses.

Preparing the slides

If new microscope slides are available, they can be used without any special treatment. However, it is more economical to reuse or recycle used microscope slides. The slides should be washed with soap and water, rinsed with water, and then rinsed with 50% aqueous methanol. The plates should be allowed to dry thoroughly on paper towels. They should be handled by the edge because fingerprints on the plate surface will make it difficult for the adsorbent to bind to the glass.

Coating the slides

The slides are coated with adsorbent by dipping them into the container of slurry. Two slides can be coated simultaneously by sandwiching them together before dipping them in the slurry. The slurry should be shaken vigorously just before dipping the slides. Since the slurry settles on standing, it should be mixed in this way before each set of slides is dipped. The depth of the slurry in the jar should be about 3 inches, and the plates should be dipped into the slurry until only about 0.25 inches at the top remains uncoated. The dipping operation should be done smoothly. The plates may be held at the top, where they will not be coated. They are dipped into the slurry and withdrawn with a slow and steady motion. The dipping operation takes about 2 seconds. Some practice may be required to get the correct timing. After dipping, the cap should be replaced on the jar, and the plates should be held for a minute until most of the solvent has evaporated. The plates may then be separated and placed on paper towels to complete the drying.

The plates should have an even coating; there should be no streaks no thin spot where glass shows through the adsorbent. The plates should not have a thick and lumpy coating. Two conditions cause thin and streaked plates. First, the slurry may not have been thoroughly mixed before the dipping operation; the adsorbent might then have settled to the bottom of the jar, and the thin slurry at the top would not have coated the slides properly. Second, the slurry simply may not have been thick enough; more silica gel G must then be added to the slurry until the consistency is proper. If the slurry is too thick, the coating on the plates will be thick, uneven, and lumpy. To correct this, slurry should be diluted with enough solvent to achieve the proper consistency. Plates with a satisfactory coating may be wiped clean with a paper towel and re-dipped. Care must be taken to handle the plates only from the top or by the sides.

Pre-prepared plates

Many manufactures supply glass plates pre-coated with a durable layer of silica gel or alumina. More conveniently, plates are also available that have either a flexible plastic backing or aluminum backing are becoming increasingly common. They are expensive, but are made quite uniformly, and being flexible, have the advantage that they do not flake easily. They can also be cut with a pair of scissors to whatever size is required.

Sample Application: Spotting the Plates

Preparing a micropipette

To apply the sample that is to be separated to the thin-layer plate, one uses a micropipette. A micropipette is easily made from a short length of thin-walled capillary tubing like that used for melting-point determinations. The capillary tubing is heated at its midpoint with a micro-burner and rotated until it is soft. When the tubing is soft, the heated portion of the tubing is drawn out until a constricted portion of tubing 4-5 cm long is formed. After cooling, the constricted portion of tubing is scored at its center with a file or a scorer and broken. The two halves yield two capillary micropipettes.

Spotting the plate

To apply a sample to the plate, begin by placing about 1 mg of a solid test substance, or one drop of a liquid test substance, in a small container like a watch glass or a test tube. Dissolve the sample in a few drops of a volatile solvent. Acetone or methylene chloride are usually suitable solvents. If a solution is to be tested, it can often be used directly. The small capillary pipet, prepared as described, is filled by dipping the pulled end into the solution to be examined. Capillary action fills the pipet. One empties the pipet by touching it lightly to the thin-layer plate at a point about 1 cm from the bottom. The spot must be high enough that it does not dissolve in the developing solvent. It is important to touch the plate very lightly and not to gouge a hole in the adsorbent. It is often helpful to blow gently on the plate as the sample is applied. This helps to keep the spot small by evaporating the solvent before it can spread out on the plate. The smaller the spot formed, the better the separation obtainable. If needed, additional material can be applied to the plate by repeating the spotting procedure. It is best to repeat to procedure with several small amounts, rather than to apply one large amount.

Developing (running) TLC Plates

Preparing a development chamber

A convenient developing chamber for microscope-slide TLC plates can be made from a 4-oz wide-mouthed screw-cap jar. The inside of the jar should be lined with a piece of filter paper, cut so that it does not quite extend around the inside of the jar. A small vertical opening (2-3 cm) should be left for observing the development. Before development, the filter paper liner inside the jar should be thoroughly moistened with the development solvent. The solvent-saturated liner helps to keep the chamber saturated with solvent vapors, there by speeding development. Once the liner is saturated, the level of solvent in the bottom of the jar is adjusted to a depth of about 5 mm, and the jar is capped and set aside until it is to be used.

Developing the TLC slide

Once the spot has been applied to the thin-layer plate and the solvent has been selected, the plate is placed in the chamber for development. The plate must be placed in the chamber carefully so that none of the coated portion touches the filter paper liner. In addition, the solvent level in the bottom of the chamber must not be above the spot that was applied to the plate, or the spotted material will dissolve in the pool of solvent instead of undergoing chromatography. Once the plate has been placed correctly, one replaces the cap on the developing chamber and waits for the solvent to advance up the plate by capillary action. This generally occurs rapidly, and one should watch carefully. As the solvent rises, the plates become visibly moist. When the solvent has advanced to within 5 mm of the coated surface, the plate should be removed, and the position of the solvent front should be marked immediately by scoring the plate along the solvent line with a pencil. The solvent front must not be allowed to travel beyond the end of the coated surface. The plate should be removed before this happens. The solvent will not actually advance beyond the end of the plate, but spots allowed to stand on a completely moistened plate on which the solvent is not in motion expand by diffusion. Once the plate has dried, any visible spots should be outlined on the plate with a pencil. If no spots are apparent, a visualization method may be needed.

Selection of a solvent for development

The development solvent used depends on the materials to be separated. One may have to try several solvents before a satisfactory separation is achieved. Since microscope slides can be prepared and developed rapidly, an empirical choice is usually not hard to make. A solvent that moves all the spotted material with the solvent front is too polar. Whereas, the solvent which does not cause any of the material in the spot to move is not polar enough.

Visualization methods

If the compounds separated by TLC are colored, it is a fortunate result, because the separation can be followed visually. More often than not, however, the compounds are colorless. The separated materials must be made visible by some reagent or some method that makes the separated compound visible. Reagent that gives rise to colored spots is called visualization reagents. Methods of viewing that make the spots apparent are visualization methods. The visualization reagent used most often is iodine. Iodine reacts with organic materials to form complexes that are either brown or yellow. The second most common method of visualization is by an ultraviolet lamp. Under UV light, compounds often look like bright spots on the plate. This often suggests the structure of the compounds, because certain types of compounds shine very brightly under UV light since they fluorescence. Another method with good results involves adding a fluorescent indicator to the adsorbent used to coat the plates. A mixture of zinc and cadmium sulfides is often used. When treated in this way and held under UV light, the entire plate fluoresces. However, dark spots appear on the plate where the separated compounds are seen to quench this fluorescence. In addition to the above methods, several chemicals methods are available that either destroy or permanently alter the separated compounds through reaction.

Most organic functional groups can be made visible if they are charred with sulfuric acid. Concentrated sulfuric acid is sprayed on the plate, which is then heated in an oven at 110 $^{\circ}$C to complete the charring.

Preparative plates

If large plates are used, materials can be separated and the separated components individually recovered from the plates. Plates used in this way are said to be preparative plates. For preparative plates, a thick layer of adsorbent is generally used. Instead of being applied as a spot or a series of the spots, the mixture to be separated is applied as line of material about 1 cm from the bottom of the plate. As the plate is developed, the separated materials form bands. After development, the separated bands are observed, usually by UV light, and the zones are outlined in pencil, if the method of visualization is destructive, most of the plate is covered with paper to protect it, and the reagent is applied only at the extreme edge of the plate. Once the zones have been identified, the adsorbent in those bands is scraped from the plate and extracted with solvent to remove the adsorbed material. Filtration removes the adsorbent, and evaporation of the solvent gives the recovered component from the mixture.

The R_f value

Thin-layer chromatography conditions include:

1. Solvent system
2. Adsorbent
3. Thickness of the adsorbent layer
4. Relative amount of material spotted

Under an established set of such conditions, a given compound always travels a fixed distance relative to the distance the solvent front travels. This ratio of the distance the compound travels to the distance the solvent front travels is called the R_f value (Figure 15.2). The symbol R_f stands for "ratio to front" and it is expressed as a decimal fraction:

$$R_f = \frac{\text{Distance travelled by substance}}{\text{Distance travelled by solvent front}}$$

When conditions of measurement are completely specified, the R_f value is constant for any given compound, and it corresponds to a physical property of that compound.

The R_f value can be used to identify an unknown compound; but like any other identification based on a single piece of data, the R_f value is best confirmed with some additional data. Many compounds can have the same R_f values, just as many different compounds have the same melting point. It is not always possible, in measuring an R_f value, to duplicate exactly the conditions of the measurement another worker used.

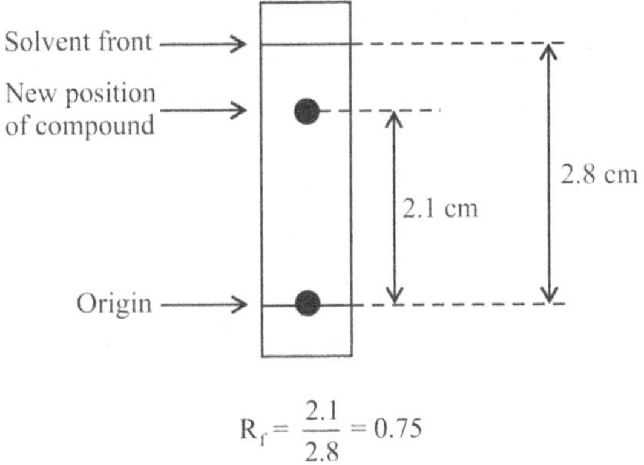

$$R_f = \frac{2.1}{2.8} = 0.75$$

Fig. 15.2 Diagrammatic representation of calculating R_f value.

Experiment 15.1

Identification of Unknown Drug by using Thin Layer Chromatography

Theory

Thin layer chromatography (TLC) is one of the methods available for the separation and tentative identification of the components presents in mixtures. A compound will travel at a rate fixed by its relative solubility in a moving solvent and stationary phase. The more soluble the component is in the solvent, the farther the component travels. The more interactions the component has with the silica gel on the thin layer plate, the less distance it will travel. The location of each component must be determined by making them visible, if they are not already visible. This may require a visualizing agent, which can be a chemical or an instrument.

The distance that the component has travelled is normally recorded by computing an R_f value (relative flow value). This value is calculated by applying the following formula:

$$R_f = \frac{\text{Distance travelled by substance}}{\text{Distance travelled by solvent front}}$$

This R_f is characteristic of the substance in the solvent system used and helps identify the unknown substance. The size of the spot provides a rough quantitative measure of the amount of the substance present. When you work with a particular group of compounds, known samples should be run with the unknown to avoid any uncertainties caused by variations in the system, as well as for comparison purposes at the time of identification.

Procedure

1. Obtain a thin layer plate. Contamination and damage to the surface of the plate may be avoided by holding the plate at the edges.

2. Using a pencil only, draw a baseline, approximately 1.5 cm from the bottom of the plate. Mark seven equidistant spots on this baseline, and label them 1, 2, 3, 4, 5, unknown and mixture.

3. Obtain six clean dry test tubes and label them using a china marker, as follows:

   Test tube 1: caffeine (a stimulant)

   Test tube 2: ibuprofen (an analgesic)

   Test tube 3: phenacetin (an analgesic)

   Test tube 4: quinine (an antimalarial)

   Test tube 5: salicylic acid (an analgesic)

   Test tube 6: unknown sample.

4. Add spatula tip full of the powdered drug in each of the labeled test tube. Be sure to avoid contamination from one tube to the next.

   Tube 6: this is an unknown sample is to be identified using the technique of thin layer chromatography.

5. In the hood, add approximately 3 mL of concentrated ammonium hydroxide to each tube, and mix gently (caution: do not inhale the ammonium hydroxide fumes). Then add 1 mL of the ethyl acetate solvent to each tube and mix thoroughly. Let the tubes stand for a few minutes in order to allow the ammonium hydroxide and ethyl acetate to separate (use a centrifuge if necessary).

6. Using a clean dropper for each tube, transfer a portion of the upper (ethyl acetate) layer to a clean, labeled tube. Be careful not to transfer any of the ammonium hydroxide layer.

7. Using a new capillary tube for each sample, spot each of the samples on the appropriate mark on the samples on the appropriate mark on the chromatography plate. Some samples may have to be spotted more than once. Let the spots dry. To the mark labeled mixture on the plate, spot one drop of each of the five standard drugs. To the mark labeled unknown the plate, spot the unknown sample from tube 6 a few times.

8. Place the plate in the prepared 'solvent chamber' located in the hood. The solvent is a mixture of ethyl acetate: methanol: ammonium hydroxide (85:10:5). When the solvent has moved ¾ of the way up the plate, remove the plate. Let it dry in the hood.

9. Examine your plate under short wavelength ultraviolet light in order to visualize your results. Be sure to check the origin for any drugs that do not readily move in the solvent.

Observations

Calculate the R_f value of each drug and identify the unknown drug.

Experiment 15.2

Identification of Amino Acids by using Thin Layer Chromatography

Theory

A mixture of Amino acids can be identified using thin layer chromatography. The position of the amino acids can be detected by spraying with ninhydrin which reacts with α-amino acids to yield highly colored products.

Chemicals required:

1. 2 % Ammonia solution.

2. 2-Propanol.

3. Ninhydrin spray: 2 % solution of ninhydrin in ethanol.

4. Separate solutions of 0.05M glycine, leucine, tyrosine in 1.5 % HCl in test tubes and an unknown sample containing three amino acids.

Procedure

1. Prepare solvent system for TLC containing 10 mL of 2% ammonia solution and 20 mL of 2-propanol in a clean TLC chamber.

2. Obtain a thin layer plate. Contamination and damage to the surface of the plate may be avoided by holding the plate at the edges.

3. Using a pencil only, draw a baseline, approximately 1.5 cm from the bottom of the plate. Mark six equidistant spots on this baseline, and label them 1, 2, 3, 4, unknown, and mixture.

4. Take four clean dry test tubes and label them using a china marker, as follows:

   Test tube 1: glycine

   Test tube 2: leucine

   Test tube 3: tyrosine

   Test tube 4: unknown sample.

5. Add spatula tip full of the powdered drug in each of the labeled test tube. Be sure to avoid contamination from one tube to the next.

   Tube 4: This is an unknown sample that you have to identify using the technique of thin layer chromatography.

6. Using a new capillary tube for each sample, spot each of the samples on the appropriate mark on the samples on the appropriate mark on the chromatography plate. Some samples may have to be spotted more than once. Let the spots dry. To the mark labeled mixture on the plate, spot one drop of each of the three standard amino acids. To the mark labeled unknown the plate, spot the unknown sample from tube 4 a few times.

7. Place the plate in the prepared 'solvent chamber' located in the hood. When the solvent has moved ¾ of the way up the plate, remove the plate. Let it dry in the hood.

8. Spray the plate with ninhydrin solution and let it dry in the hood.

9. Place the plate in an oven at 100-110 °C for about 10 min, or until the spots appear on the plate.

Observations

Calculate the R_f value of each amino acid and identify the unknown amino acid by visual comparison of spot colors and by comparing the R_f values.

$$R_f = \frac{\text{Distance travelled by substance}}{\text{Distance travelled by solvent front}}$$

CHAPTER 16

Column Chromatography

Column chromatography is one of the most useful methods for the separation and purification of both solids and liquids. The principle of column chromatography is based on differential adsorption of substance by the adsorbent. It is used to purify individual chemical compounds from mixtures of compounds. It is often used for preparative applications on scales from micrograms up to kilograms.

Apparatus

Columns can be as thin as a pencil to a diameter of several feet in industrial processes. They can separate milligram to kilogram quantities of materials. In this experiment, approximately 50 mg of mixture can be separated so that small column is required. Figure 16.1 shows the typical set-up. It is essential to have several clean tared Erlenmeyer flasks, reaction tubes, beakers, test tubes or vials available to collect the solvent and compounds as they elute. Once the general set-up ready packing of the stationary phase in the column can be initiated.

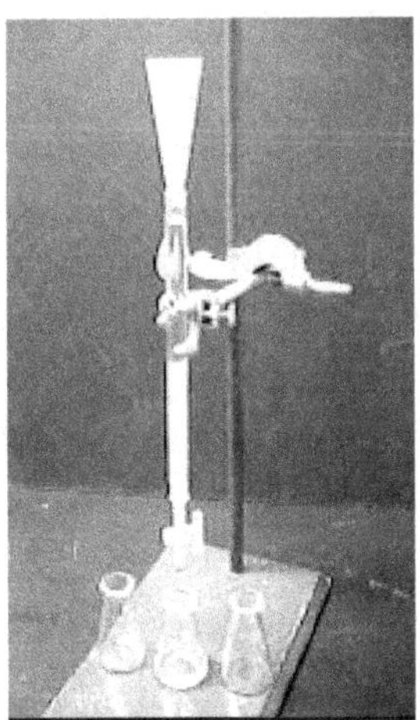

Fig. 16.1 Typical micro scale column chromatography setup.

Absorbents used

Column chromatography is a technique based on both absorptivity and solubility. It is a solid-liquid phase-partitioning technique. The solid may be almost any material that does not dissolve in the associated liquid phase. The usual adsorbents employed in column chromatography are silica, alumina, calcium carbonate, calcium phosphate, magnesia, starch, etc; selection of solvent is based on the nature of both the solvent and the adsorbent.

Principle of Column Chromatography

If adsorbent is added to a solution containing mixture of compounds, some of these compounds will get adsorbed onto the surface of adsorbent. Various kinds of forces exist between adsorbent and compounds to be adsorbed. Non-polar compounds binds to the adsorbent using weak Van der Waals forces, rendering the molecules to bind weakly to the adsorbent unless compound is of high molecular weight. Polar compounds bind through stronger forces like, dipole-dipole interaction, co-ordination and hydrogen bonding.

Similarly, polar solvents dissolve polar molecules and non-polar solvents dissolve non-polar molecules. Thus, the extent to which any solvent can wash an adsorbed compound from adsorbent depends on the polarity of the solvent.

In column chromatography, mixture to be separated is introduced onto the top of a cylindrical glass column packed with adsorbent. The adsorbent (stationary phase) is then continuously washed by a solvent (mobile phase) passing through the column. Initially, the mixture to be separated is at the top of the column. The continuous flow of solvent through the column elutes/washes them down the column **(Figure 16.2)**. As the solutes pass down the column to fresh adsorbent, new equilibria are established between the adsorbent, solute and solvent. Due to this constant equilibration, different compounds move down the column at different rates depending upon their relative affinity for the adsorbent on one hand and solvent on the other.

As the components of the mixture are separated, they begin to form moving bands, each band containing a single component. If the column is long enough and the various other parameters are correctly chosen, the bands separate from one another, leaving gaps of pure solvent in between. As each band passes out the bottom of the column, it can be collected completely before the next band arrives.

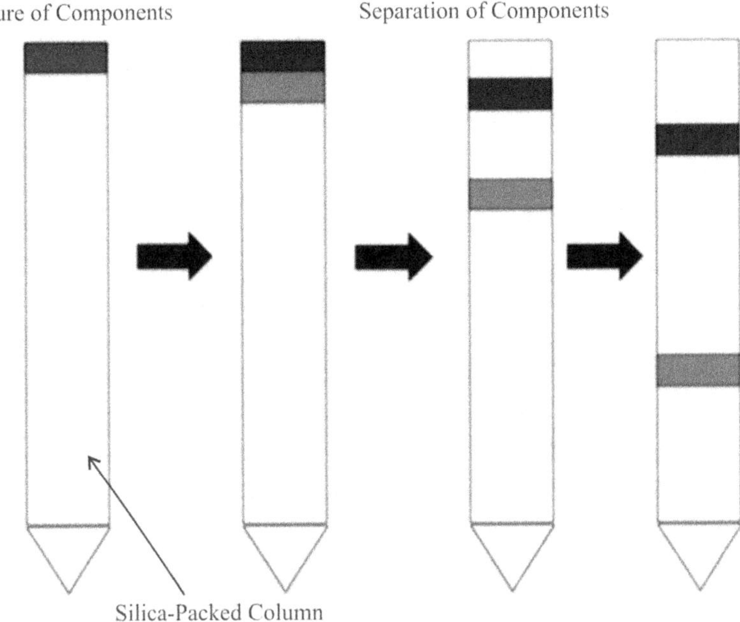

Fig. 16.2 Elution of components down the column.

Parameters affecting separation

Chromatography is truly a sophisticated method of separating mixtures. Its versatility results from the many factors that can be adjusted. These include:

1. Adsorbent chosen.

2. Polarity of solvent or solvent chosen.

3. Size of column (both length and diameter) relative to amount of material to be chromatographed.

Rate of elution or flow

By careful choice of conditions, almost any mixture can be separated. Two fundamental choices for anyone attempting a chromatographic separation are the kind of adsorbent and the solvent system. In general, non-polar compounds pass through the column faster than polar compounds, since they have a smaller affinity for the adsorbent. If the adsorbent chosen binds all the solute molecules (both polar and non polar), they will not move down the column. On the other hand, if a too polar solvent is chosen, all the solutes (polar and non polar) may simply be washed through the column, with no separation taking place. The adsorbent and the solvent should be chosen so that neither is excessively favored in the equilibrium competition for solute molecules.

1. Adsorbents

The choice of adsorbent often depends on the types of compounds to be separated. Cellulose, starch and sugars are used for poly-functional plant and animal materials (natural products) very sensitive to acid base interactions. Magnesium silicate is often used for separating acetylated sugars, steroids and essential oils. Silica gel and florisil are relatively mild towards most compounds and are widely used for a variety of functional group - hydrocarbons, alcohols, ketones, esters, acids, azo-compounds and amines.

2. Solvents

Sometimes a single solvent can be found that will separate all the component of a mixture. Sometimes a mixture of solvents can be found that will achieve separation. More often, one must start elution with a non polar solvent to remove relatively non-polar compounds from the column and then gradually increase the solvent polarity to force compounds of greater polarity to come down the column or elute (Table 16.1). When the polarity of the solvent has to be changed during a chromatographic separation, some precautions must be taken. Rapid changes from one solvent to another are to be avoided (especially when silica gel or alumina are involved). Usually small percentage of a new solvent is mixed slowly into the one in use until the percentage reaches the desired level. If this is not done, the column packing often cracks as a result of the heat liberated when alumina or silica gel is mixed with a solvent. The solvent solvates the adsorbent and the formation of a weak bond generates heat.

Table 16.1 Solvents for chromatography.

Petroleum ether	
Cyclohexane	
Carbon tetrachloride*	
Benzene*	
Chloroform*	
Methylene chloride	
Diethyl ether	Increasing polarity and solvent power towards polar functional groups
Ethyl acetate	
Acetone	
Pyridine	
Ethanol	
Methanol	
Water	
Acetic acid	

*Suspected carcinogens

1. Column size and adsorbent quantity

The column size and the amount of adsorbent must also be selected correctly to separate a given amount of sample efficiently. As a rule of thumb, the amount of adsorbent should be 25-30 times, by weight, the amount of material to be separated by chromatography. Additionally the column should have a height to diameter ratio about 8:1.

2. Flow rate

The rate at which solvent flows through the column is also significant in the effectiveness of the separation. In general, the time the mixture to be separated remains on the column is directly proportional to the extent of equilibration between stationary and moving phases. Thus, similar compounds eventually separate if they remain on the column long enough. The time a material remains on the column depends on the flow rate of the solvent. If the flow is too slow, however, the substances in the mixture, when they are in the solvent, may diffuse faster than the rate at which they move down the column. Then the bands grow wider and more diffuse and the separation becomes poorer.

Packing the Column: Typical Problems

The most critical operation in column chromatography is packing (filling with adsorbent) the column. The column of alumina (or other solid adsorbent), the column packing, must be evenly packed and free of irregularities, air bubbles and gaps. As a compound travel down the column, it moves in an advancing zone, or band. It is important that the leading edge, or front, of this band be horizontal or perpendicular to the long axis of the column. First, if the top surface edge of the adsorbent packing is not level, non horizontal bands result. Second, bands may also be non horizontal if the column is not held in an exactly vertical position in both planes (front to back and side to side).

Methods of packing

1. *Dry method:* In this method the column is first filled with dry stationary phase powder up to the desired length, followed by the addition of mobile phase, which is flushed through the column until it is completely wet and from this point is never allowed to run dry.

2. *Wet method:* In this method, slurry is prepared of the eluent with the stationary phase powder and then carefully poured into the column. Care must be taken to avoid air bubbles. A solution of the organic material is pipetted on top of the stationary phase. This layer is usually topped with a small layer of sand or with cotton or glass wool to protect the shape of the organic layer from the velocity of newly added eluent. Eluent is slowly passed through the column to advance the organic material. Often a spherical eluent reservoir or an eluent-filled and stopped separating funnel put on top of the column.

Applying the sample to the column

The solvent (or solvent mixture) used to pack the column is normally the least polar elution solvent; one intends to use during the chromatography. For the best separation, the compound is applied to the top of the column, undiluted if it is a liquid, or in a very small amount of a highly polar solvent if it is a solid. Once the sample has been properly applied, the level surface of the adsorbent may be protected by carefully filling the top of the column with solvent and sprinkling clean, white sand into the column so as to form a small protective layer on top of the adsorbent.

Elution techniques

Solvents for analytical and preparative chromatography should be pure reagents. One usually begins elution of the products with a non polar solvent, like hexane or petroleum ether. The polarity of the elution solvent can be increased gradually by adding successively greater percentages of either ether or toluene (for instance 1%, 2%, 5%, 10%, 50%) or some other solvent of greater solvent power (polarity) than hexane. The flow of solvent through the column should not be too rapid or the solutes will not have time to equilibrate with the adsorbent as they pass down the column. If the rate of flow is too low or stopped for a period, diffusion can become a problem - the solute band will diffuse or spread out, in all directions. As a general rule (and only an approximate one), most columns are run with flow rates ranging from 5 to 50 drops of effluent per minute.

Recovering the separated compounds

In recovering each of the separated compounds of a chromatographic separation when they are solids, the various correct fractions are combined, evaporated and recrystallised. If the compounds are liquids, the correct fractions are combined, evaporated and distilled. The combination of chromatography - crystallisation or chromatography - distillation usually yields very pure compounds.

Column chromatography is an extremely time consuming stage in any lab and can quickly become the bottleneck for any process lab. Therefore, several manufacturers like Teledyne Isco, have developed automated flash chromatography systems (typically referred to as LPLC, low pressure liquid chromatography, around 350-525 kPa or 51-76.1 psi) that minimize human involvement in the purification process. Automated systems will include components normally found on more expensive high performance liquid chromatography (HPLC) systems such as a gradient pump, sample injection ports, a UV detector and a fraction collector to collect the eluent. Typically these automated systems can separate samples from a few milligrams up to an industrial many kilogram scale and offer a much cheaper and quicker solution to doing multiple injections on prep-HPLC systems.

Advantages of column chromatography

1. Relatively low cost.

2. Disposability of the stationary phase used in the process which prevents cross-contamination and stationary phase degradation due to recycling.

Experiment 16.1

To Separate Organic Compounds with the help of Column Chromatographic Technique

Theory

The rate at which the components of a mixture are separated depends on the activity of the adsorbent and polarity of the solvent. If the activity of the adsorbent is very high and polarity of the solvent is very low, then the separation is very slow but gives a good separation. On the other hand, if the activity of adsorbent is low and polarity of the solvent is high the separation is rapid but gives only a poor separation, i.e., the component separated is not 100% pure.

The adsorbent is made into slurry with a suitable liquid and placed in a cylindrical tube that is plugged at the bottom by a piece of glass wool or porous disc. The mixture to be separated is dissolved in a suitable solvent and introduced at the top of the column and is allowed to pass through the column. As the mixture moves down through the column, the components are adsorbed at different regions depending on their ability for adsorption. The component with greater adsorption power will be adsorbed at the top and the other will be adsorbed at the bottom. The different components can be desorbed and collected separately by adding more solvent at the top and this process is known as *elution*. That is, the process of dissolving out of the components from the adsorbent is called elution and the solvent is called eluent. The weakly adsorbed component will be eluted more rapidly than the other. The different fractions are collected separately. Distillation or evaporation of the solvent from the different fractions gives the pure components.

Chemicals required

1. *p*-nitrophenol and *o*-nitrophenol mixture to be chromatographed

2. Silica gel for column chromatography

3. Petroleum ether

Procedure

1. Preparation of the Column

(i)   Place the column in a ring stand in a vertical position.

(ii) A plug of glass wool is pushed down to the bottom of the column.

(iii) Prepare slurry of silica gel with a suitable solvent and pour gently into the column.

(iv) Open the stop cock and allow some solvent to drain out. The layer of solvent should always cover the adsorbent; otherwise cracks will develop in the column.

2. Adding the Sample to the Column

(i)   Dissolve the sample mixture in a minimum amount of solvent (petroleum ether).

(ii) Remove the solvent by placing the mixture in a rotary evaporator at a low temperature.

(iii) Place the dry powder on a piece of weighing paper and transfer it to the top of the column through the funnel.

3. Developing the Chromatogram

(i)   Attach a dropping funnel filled with petroleum ether on to the column.

(ii) Add petroleum ether continuously from the funnel to the top of the column.

(iii) Open the stopcock carefully.

(iv) The components of the mixture run down the column forming two separate yellow bands.

4. Recovering the Constituents

(i)   Continue running the petroleum ether till both the bands is eluted out separately.

(ii) Collect the constituents in two different round bottomed flasks. (*ortho*-nitrophenol is obtained first, followed by *para*-nitro phenol.).

(iii) Evaporate the solvent by placing the mixture in a rotary evaporator.

Experiment 16.2

To Separate Mixture of Dye with the help of Column Chromatographic Technique

Material required

1. Methylene blue (MW = 373.90 gm/mol)

2. Methyl orange (MW = 327.34 gm/mol)

3. Ethyl alcohol

4. Water

5. Alumina 90

Procedure

Pack a conventional size chromatography column with activated alumina. Use a glass wool plug in the bottom. The column has a clamp to stop the flow of the solvent. Mix 10 mL ethanol and 10 gm alumina to obtain slurry. Fill this slurry to the column and wait until alumina settles down to 4-5 cm height.

1. Always keep some ethanol above the top of the alumina. Newer allow the alumina to be dry. Allow the ethanol to come to about 1 mm at the top of the column and stopper the bottom of the column with a hose clamp.

2. Add a mixture prepared with 0.6 mL methylene blue and 0.4 mL methyl orange which have the same concentration, 0.25 mg/mL. Introduce gently 1 mL dye solution onto the top of the column.

3. Carefully add about 10 ml of ethanol to the column and allow it to drip through. Collect uncolored eluent in the waste, but as soon as the colored compound begins to emerge, collect this in a beaker. Record the time to reach first dye drop.

4. Record the rate of movement of colored rings through the packing.

5. When the first dye is either completely or nearly emerged from the column, add 10 mL of water carefully to the top of the column. Once again, collect clear eluent in the waste. The second dye should be collected in a separate beaker.

6. Note the volume of each of the two dye solutions. If they are too dark, they may need to be diluted.

7. To do this, take 1 mL of the solution and carefully dilute it to 5 or 10 mL with the eluent in a clean tube.

Observation and Calculation

Using UV Spectrophotometer, find the concentrations of the dye solutions. Plotting absorbance versus concentration of standard solutions, draw the calibration lines. The calibration lines for methylene blue and methyl orange should be drawn at 650 nm and 450 nm respectively.

CHAPTER 17

Colorimetry

The term *colorimetry* originates from the times when measurements were done by comparing the color of a component under investigation with a standard color by the eye. While this principle is still the basis of modern techniques, of course the measurement with the eye has been replaced by the measurement of photons with a photon detector in order to eliminate experimental errors.

A colorimetric method often gives more accurate results at low concentrations than the corresponding titrimetric analysis and is simpler to carry out. This method can be certainly applied in some conditions where conventional titrimetric experiments do not exist e.g., for the determination of biological substances.

Principle of Colorimeter

Measurement of absorbance (A)

Unknown compounds may be identified by their characteristic absorption spectra in the ultraviolet, visible or infrared regions. Enzyme-catalyzed reactions frequently can be followed by measuring spectrophoto-metrically the appearance of a product or disappearance of a substrate. A spectrophotometer/colorimeter is an instrument for measuring the absorbance of a solution by measuring the amount of light of a given wavelength that is transmitted by a sample.

Light and spectrum profile

Light can be categorized according to its wavelength. Light in the short wavelengths of 200 to 400 nm is referred to as ultraviolet (UV). Light in the longer wavelengths of 700 to 900 nm is referred to as near infrared (near IR).

Beer-Lambert law

The Beer-Lambert law states that the amount of light absorbed is proportional to the number of molecules of absorbing substance in the light path, i.e., absorption is proportional both to the concentration of the sample solution and to the length of the light path through the solution. This relationship can be expressed as follows:

Absorbance, A= $\varepsilon \times c \times l$

where   c = concentration of the sample (in Moles/liter),

      l = path length of light passing through the solution (in cm)

      ε = molar extinction coefficient

To determine the absolute concentration of a pure substance, a standard curve is constructed from the known concentrations and using that standard curve, the absorbance reading of the unknown concentration was determined. The determination of unknown concentration from the standard curve is done by drawing a line parallel to the X-axis from the point on the Y axis that corresponds to the absorbance of the unknown. This line will be made to intersect the standard curve drawn and is extended vertically such that it meets the X-axis and the concentration of unknown is read from the X-axis.

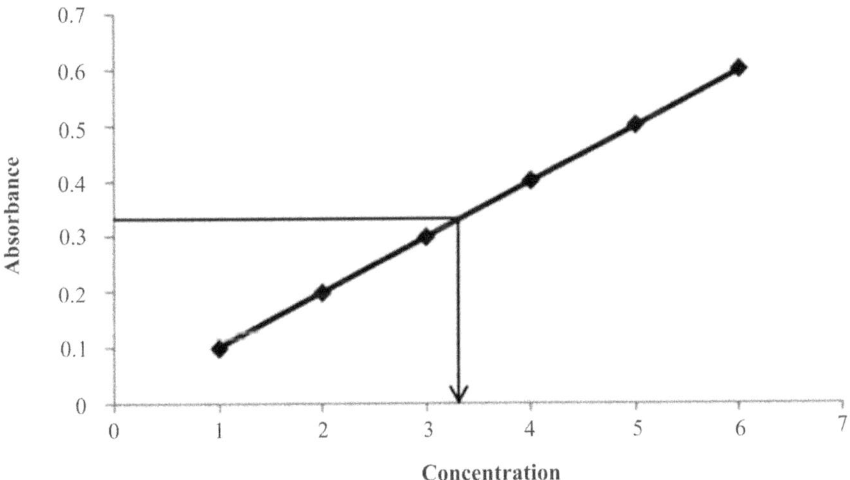

Colorimetric analysis should satisfy following criteria

1. ***Specificity to the color reaction:*** A few reactions are specific for a particular substance but many gives color for a small group of similar substances i.e., they are selective. Specificity of the reaction may be obtained by introducing complex-forming substances, altering the oxidation state or controlling the pH.

2. ***Proportionality between color and concentration:*** In case of visual colorimeters, it is important that the color intensity of a solution increases linearly with concentration of the substance.

3. ***Stability of the color:*** The color produced should be stable in order to permit an accurate reading. This applies to those reactions in which color intensifies with time.

4. ***Reproducibility:*** The colorimetric method used should be reproducible under given experimental conditions.

5. ***Clarity of the solution:*** The solution under experiment should be free from any kind of turbidity or precipitation as it scatters light.

6. ***High sensitivity:*** The color reaction should be highly sensitive in order to determine very small amount of the substance and the reaction product should absorb strongly in visible region.

Experiment 17.1

To Determine Amount of Amino Acids using Colorimetry

Theory

Amino acids are known as the building blocks of all proteins. There are 20 different amino acids commonly found in proteins. Amino acids comprise of a carboxyl group and an amino group attached to the same carbon atom (α carbon). They vary in size, structure, electric charge and solubility in water because of the variation in their side chains (R groups). Thus detection, quantification and identification of amino acids in any sample constitute an important step in the study of proteins. Alpha amino acids react with Ninhydrin involved in the development of color which is explained by the following five steps.

$$\text{Alpha-amino acid} + \text{Ninhydrin} \longrightarrow \text{Reduced ninhydrin} + \text{Alpha amino acid} + H_2O$$

This is an oxidative deamination reaction that elicits two hydrogen atoms from the alpha amino acid to produce alpha-imino acid. Also the ninhydrin reduced and loses an oxygen atom with the formation of water molecule.

$$\text{Alpha-amino acid} + H_2O \longrightarrow \text{alpha-keto acid} + NH_3$$

The rapid hydrolysis of NH group in the alpha-imino acid will cause the formation of an alpha-keto acid with an ammonia molecule. This alpha-keto acid is further involved in the decaroxylation reaction of step.

$$\text{Alpha-keto acid} + NH_3 \longrightarrow \text{Aldehyde} + CO_2$$

Under a heated condition to form an aldehyde that has one less carbon atom than the original amino acid. Carbon dioxide molecule is produced along with aldehyde. These first three steps produce the reduced ninhydrin and ammonia that are required for the production of color .The overall reaction for the above reactions is simply explained in Reaction as follows:

$$\text{Alpha-amino acid} + 2\ \text{Ninhydrin} \longrightarrow CO_2 + \text{aldehyde} +$$
$$\text{final complex(BLUE)} + 3\,H_2O$$

In summary, ninhydrin, which is originally yellow, reacts with amino acid and turns deep purple. It is this purple color that is detected in this method. Ninhydrin will react with a free alpha-amino group, NH_2-C-COOH. This group is present in all amino acids, proteins or peptides. Whereas, the decarboxylation reaction will proceed for a free amino acid, it will not happen for peptides and proteins. The primary amino groups react with ninhydrin to form the purple color dye now called Ruhemann's purple (RP) was discovered by Siegfried Ruhemann in 1910. In the quantitative estimation of amino acid using Ninhydrin reagent, the absorbance of the Ruhemann's purple formed by the reaction at 570 nm is measured.

Chemicals required

1. Standard amino acid stock solution: 150 micrograms of Standard amino acid stock solution (150 µg/mL).

2. 0.2M Acetate buffer (pH=5.5).

3. 8% w/v of Ninhydrin reagent: Weigh 8 g of ninhydrin and dissolve in 100 mL of acetone.

4. 50% v/v ethanol.

5. Distilled water.

Procedure

1. Pipette out different volumes (0.1-1 mL) of standard amino acid solution to the respective labeled test tubes.

2. Add distilled water in all the test tubes to make up the volume to 4 mL.

3. Add 4 mL of distilled water to the test tube labeled Blank.

4. Now add 1 mL of ninhydrin reagent to all the test tubes including the test tubes labeled 'blank' and 'unknown'.

5. Mix the contents of the tubes by vortexing/shaking the tubes.

6. Put a few marble chips in each tube.

7. Cover the mouth of the tubes with aluminium foil.

8. Place all the test tubes in boiling water bath for 15 minutes.

9. Cool the test tubes in cold water and add 1mL of ethanol to each test tube and mix well.

10. Now record the absorbance at 570 nm of each solution using a colorimeter.

Observation and Calculations

Plot a calibration curve between absorbance and concentration (Figure 17.1) of the standard amino acid. Read out the concentration of unknown sample from this curve.

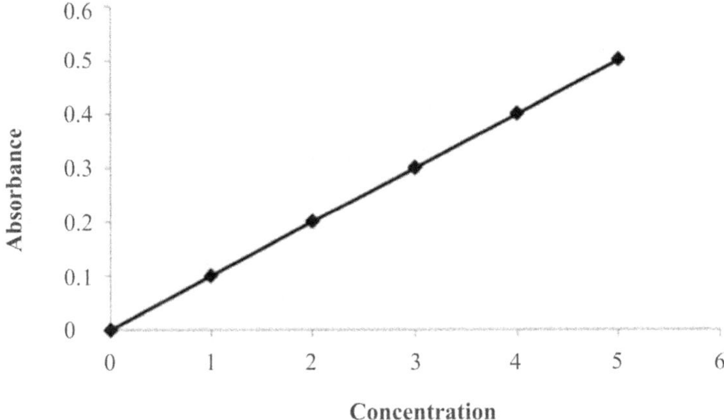

Fig. 17.1 Calibration curve.

Experiment 17.2

To Determine Amount of Blood Glucose Level using Colorimetry

Theory

Glucose is a simple sugar which is a permanent and immediate primary source of energy to all the cells in our body. The glucose in blood is obtained from the food. This glucose gets absorbed by intestines and distributed to all of the cells in body through bloodstream and breaks it down for energy. Body tries to maintain a constant supply of glucose for cells by maintaining a constant blood glucose concentration. The concentration of glucose in blood, expressed in mg/dl, is defined by the term glycemia. The value of blood sugar in humans generally ranges from 70-110 mg/dl. Blood sugar levels are regulated by the hormones insulin and glucagon which act antagonistically. Glucose oxidase is an enzyme extracted from the growth medium of *Aspergillus niger*. Glucose oxidase catalyze the oxidation of β-*D*-glucose present in the plasma to *D*-glucono-1,5-lactone with the formation of hydrogen peroxide; the lactone is then slowly hydrolyzed to *D*-gluconic acid. The hydrogen peroxide produced is then broken down to oxygen and water by a peroxidase enzyme. Oxygen then react with an oxygen acceptor such as *ortho*-toluidine which itself converted to a colored compound, the amount of which can be measured colorimetrically.

Materials required

1. *Collection of blood sample:* About 2 mL of patient's blood collected by venipuncture into a tube containing a mixture of ethylene-diaminetetraacetic acid and sodium fluoride in the ratio of 1:2 (W/W). Five mg of the mixture is adequate for 2 mL of blood. The tube should be thoroughly shaken for complete mixing.

Preparation of anticoagulant mixture: 100 mg of EDTA and 20 mg of sodium fluoride should be mixed and ground into a fine powder using a blender. This should preferably do in a fume hood. The mixture should be stored in a clean container.

Reagents

1. 2N Sodium hydroxide (NaOH): 8 g of NaOH is dissolve and finally make up the volume to 100 mL with distilled water.

2. Sodium Sulphate-Zinc sulphate reagent: Dilute 55 mL of the zinc sulphate solution (10g/100 mL $ZnSO_4.7H_2O$) to 1 liter with the sodium sulphate solution (93 mmol/liter).

3. Phosphate buffer 0.05M pH-7.2

4. ***Glucose oxidase reagent:*** Freshly prepare this reagent by dissolving 25 mg of glucose oxidase and 1% *o*-toluidine in the sodium phosphate buffer. Add a small quantity of peroxidase (2 mg) and makeup to 250 mL with the buffer. This solution is active for about 4 weeks if stored in a brown colored bottle at 4 $^{\circ}$C.

Procedure

1. ***Preparation of Test:*** Pipette 0.1 mL of blood into 1.8 mL of sodium sulphate-zinc sulphate reagent in a centrifuge tube. Add 0.1 mL of 2N sodium hydroxide, centrifuge at 3000 rpm for 5 minutes and take 0.5 mL of supernatant in duplicate.

2. ***Preparation of Blank:*** Take 0.5 mL of distilled water.

3. ***Preparation of Standard:*** Prepare standard concentration of glucose (200 mg/dl), use 0.5 mL of a range of glucose solutions (50 mg/dl, 100 mg/dl, 150 mg/dl and 200 mg/dl) suitably diluted from standard.

    (a) 50 mg/dl – 125 µl glucose standard + 375 µl distilled water
    (b) 100 mg/dl – 250 µl glucose standard + 250 µl distilled water
    (c) 150 mg/dl – 375 µl glucose standard + 125 µl distilled water
    (d) 200 mg/dl – 500 µl glucose standard

4. Add 5 mL of the glucose oxidase reagent, incubate for 1 h at 37 $^{\circ}$C and read the extinction at 540 nm against the reagent blank.

5. If the absorbance reading of the sample is too high, dilute the supernatant which was obtained earlier, 2x with distilled water and repeat the subsequent step.

Observation

Construct a calibration curve (Figure 17.2) by plotting the absorbance on the y-axis and the concentration on the x-axis. From this curve, the absorbance reading of any sample can be converted into concentration.

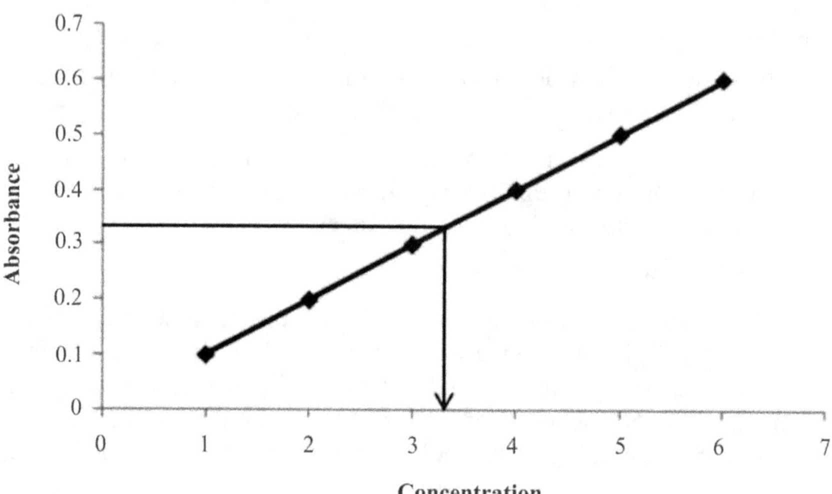

Fig. 17.2 Calibration curve.

CHAPTER 18

Spectroflurometry

Fluorometry or spectrofluorometry, is a type of electromagnetic spectroscopy which analyses fluorescence from a sample. It involves using a beam of light, usually ultraviolet light, that excites the electrons in molecules of certain compound and causes them to emit light of a lower energy, typically, but not necessarily, visible light. A complementary technique is an absorption spectroscopy. Devices that measures fluorescence are called fluorimeters.

Molecules have various states referred to as energy levels. Fluorescence spectroscopy is primarily concerned with electronic and vibrational states. Generally, the species being examined will have a ground electronic state (a low energy state) of interest and an excited electronic state of higher energy. Within each of these electronic states are various vibrational states.

In fluorescence spectroscopy, the species is first excited, by absorbing a photon, from its ground electronic state to one of the various vibrational states in the excited electronic state. Collisions with other molecules cause the excited molecule to loose vibrational energy until it reaches the lowest vibrational state of the excited electronic state.

The molecule then drops down to one of the various vibrational levels of the ground electronic state again, emitting a photon in the process. As molecule may drop down into any of several vibrational levels in the ground state, the emitted photons will have different energies, and thus frequencies. Therefore, by analyzing the different frequencies of light emitted in fluorescent spectroscopy, along with their relative intensities, the structure of the different vibrational levels can be determined.

In a typical experiment, the different frequencies of fluorescent light emitted by a sample are measured, holding the excitation light at a constant wavelength. This is called an emission spectrum. An excitation spectrum is measured by recording a number of emission spectra using different wavelengths of excitation light.

Experiment 18.1

Determination of Riboflavin by using Spectrofluorometry

Theory

Riboflavin is an important vitamin of the B complex (vitamin B_{12}) acting as an intermediary in the transfer of the electrons in biological redox reactions and having an important function in cell growth. As with all vitamins of the B complex, riboflavin is only synthesized by microorganisms and higher vegetables, not by animals, which must obtain it from their food. Considering the high concentrations of B complex vitamins present in meat and milk, these foods are the best natural sources of riboflavin in human diet. In many applications, minimum sample treatment required because the native fluorescence properties of the analyte are used. For cases in which the analyte is not fluorescent or the fluorescence quantum efficiency is inadequate, derivatization reactions are used to convert the analyte into a product with good fluorescence characteristics. The fluorescence signal of the product is related to the analyte concentration. Most commonly, the analytical reaction is allowed to reach equilibrium before measurements are made.

In this experiment, prepare an accurate calibration curve of fluorescence intensity versus known concentration of riboflavin. These calibration curves will then be used to determine the concentration of a riboflavin solution prepared.

Chemicals required

1. Riboflavin (solid)
2. 10 µg/mL Riboflavin standard
3. 1 % (v/v) acetic acid
4. Unknown vitamin tablet

Procedure

1. Using the stock riboflavin solution containing 10 μg/mL of riboflavin, prepare a series of ten standard solutions by dilutions with 1% (v/v) acetic acid solution.

2. The strongest standard should not contain more than 1 μg/mL of riboflavin.

3. The weakest standard solution should contain less than 0.1 μg/mL of riboflavin.

4. Set the excitation wavelength at 444 nm and emission wavelength at 520 nm.

5. Take the fluorescent intensity of each standard dilution against the blank.

6. Weigh accurately 30 tablets and powder them.

7. Prepare a solution by dissolving a weighed amount of powder equivalent to about 10 mg of riboflavin in 100 mL of 1% acetic acid solution.

8. Similarly, record the fluorescence intensity of the sample solution and determine the concentration of riboflavin in μg/mL.

Observation and Calculation

Plot a calibration curve by plotting a graph between the concentration and emission intensity. Read out the concentration of unknown solution from the calibration curve. Multiply with dilution factor to get the concentration in the sample.

Experiment 18.2

Determination of Thiamine by using Spectrofluorometry

Theory

Thiamine, also known as vitamin B_1 and aneurine hydrochloride, is the term for a family of molecules sharing a common structural feature responsible for its activity as a vitamin. It is one of the B vitamins. Its most common form is a colorless chemical compound with chemical formula $C_{12}H_{17}N_4OS$. Its chemical structure contains a pyrimidine ring and a thiazole ring. This form of thiamin is soluble in water, methanol, and glycerol and practically insoluble in acetone, ether, chloroform and benzene.

It is a non-fluorescent compound but can be assayed by fluorimetric method. It is quantitatively converted into fluorescent compound, thiochrome by alkaline potassium ferricyanide. The thiochrome (biologically inactive) is estimated by fluorimetric method.

Chemicals required

1. **Potassium ferricyanide ($K_3Fe(CN)_6$) solution:** Dissolve 1.0 g of the substance in 100 mL of water. Now mix 4 mL of the $K_3Fe(CN)_6$ solution with sufficient 15% w/v NaOH to make 100 mL of oxidizing reagent

2. **Thiamine HCl stock solution:** Transfer 25 mg of thiamine HCl to a 100 mL volumetric flask. Dissolve this in 3000 mL of 20% C_2H_5OH which has been adjusted with 3N HCl to a pH of 4.0. Now, add the acidified alcohol to make up the volume.

Procedure

1. To make the assay preparation, place in a suitable volumetric flask sufficient powder from the tablets to be assayed, such that when diluted to volume with 0.2N HCl, the resulting solution will contain about 100 mg of thiamine HCl per mL.

2. Now dilute 5 mL of this solution quantitatively and stepwise using 0.2N HCl to an estimated concentration of 0.2 mg of thiamine HCl/mL.

3. Prepare the standard preparation by diluting a portion of the stock solution, quantitatively and stepwise with, 0.2N HCl to obtain a preparation of 0.2 mg of thiamine HCl/mL.

4. The next step is to take three test tubes of about 40 mL capacity and pipette 5 mL of the standard preparation while quickly (within 2 seconds) adding 3 mL of the oxidizing reagent and 20 mL of isobutyl alcohol, mixing by vigorous shaking.

5. Now prepare a blank of the standard preparation in fourth test tube by substituting for the oxidizing agent an equal volume of the 15 % NaOH and proceeding in the same manner.

6. Repeat this procedure on the standard preparation with the assay preparation by taking 3 test tubes, including the making of a blank.

7. Next, into each of eight test tubes, add 2 mL of 100% C_2H_5OH and allow the phases to separate.

8. Decant to draw off 10 mL of the clear supernatant isobutyl alcohol solution into standardized cells.

9. Then measure the fluorescence in a suitable fluorometer having an input filter of narrow transmittance range with a maximum of 365 nm and an output filter with a maximum of about 465 nm.

Calculation

Calculate the mg of thiamine HCl in each 5 mL of the assay preparation using the formula:

$$\frac{A-b}{S-d}$$

In which A and S are the average flurometer reading of the portion of the assay and standard preparation treated with the oxidizing reagent and b and d are the readings of the blanks of the assay preparation and standard preparation respectively.

CHAPTER 19

UV/Visible Spectroscopy

UV/ Visible Spectroscopy

The technique of ultraviolet-visible spectroscopy is one of the most frequently employed in pharmaceutical analysis and the instrument which measure the ratio or a function of the ratio of the intensity of two beams of light in the ultraviolet/visible region is called UV/Visible spectrophotometer.

Principle and theory of UV/Visible spectroscopy

Ultraviolet spectra arise from transition of electron within a molecule or ion, from lower to a higher electronic energy level. When a molecule or ion absorb up radiation of frequency υ sec^{-1}, the electron in that molecule undergoes transition from lower to a higher energy level or molecule orbital, the energy difference is given by:

$$E = h\,\upsilon\ erg$$

Various types of transitions that take place in molecule are as follows:

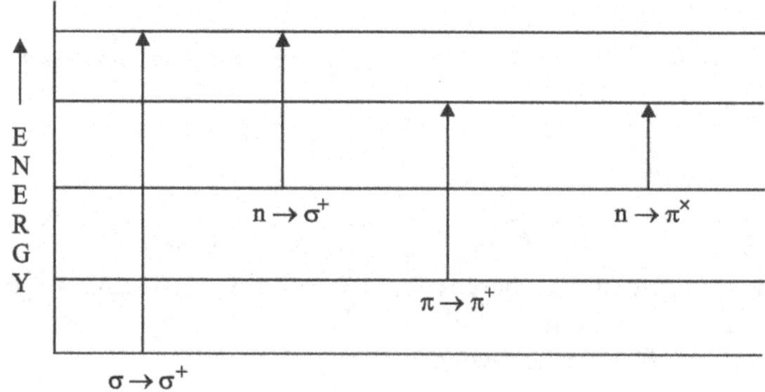

Fig. 19.1 Electron excitation-energies.

order:

$$n \longrightarrow \pi^* < \pi \longrightarrow \pi^* < n \longrightarrow \sigma^* < \sigma$$

Fundamental law of photometry

The radiant power of a beam of radiation is proportional to the number of photons per unit time. Absorption occurs when photons collide with a molecule and raise the molecule to some excited state. Each molecule can be thought of as having a cross-sectional area for photon capture and photon must pass within this area to interact with the molecule. The rate of absorption as a beam of photons passes through a medium depends on the number of photon collisions with absorbing atoms or molecules per unit time.

If the number of absorbing molecule is doubled by doubling either the length of the path of radiation through the medium or the concentration of absorbing species, the rate of absorption of photon doubles. Likewise, doubling the beam power doubles the number of photons that pass through the medium in unit time and doubles the number of collisions with absorbing molecules in limited time when the number of absorbing molecule remains constant (Willard, 2003).

Beer-Lambert's Law

After passing of light through a transparent cell containing light absorbing solution the reduction in the intensity of light may occur due to reflection at the inner and outer surface of the cells, scatter by particles in the solution and absorption of light by a molecule in solution. These former two factors can be compensated by using a reference cell and filtration of solution (Guelbaut, 1963; Beckett, 2005).

The intensity of light absorbed is given by:

$$I_{absorbed} = i_0 - i_t$$

where,

i_0 = original intensity of incident light

i_t = intensity of transmitted light.

Lambert in 1760 state that rate of decrease in the intensity of light with thickness b, of a medium is proportional to the intensity of incident light, expressed mathematically as,

$$-di/db \propto i$$

After integration and conversion to common logarithm, expression becomes,

$$\text{Log } i_0 / i_t = k'b / 2.303$$

where,

k' is called as proportionality constant

So, Lambert law is defined as intensity of a beam of parallel monochromatic radiation decrease exponentially as it passes through a medium of homogenous thickness.

Beer's law state that intensity of a beam of parallel monochromatic radiation decreases exponentially with the concentration of solution is expressed as:

$$-di/dc \propto i,$$

$$\log i_0/i_t = k'' c/2.303$$

where,

k'' is called as proportionality constant.

So after combination of these laws yields the Beer's Lambert's law was expressed as:

$$A = \log i_0 / i_t = \varepsilon bc$$

In which proportionality constant $k'/2.303$ and $k''/2.303$ are combined as a single constant called as absorptivity constant the units of absorptivity constant is mol dm^{-3} cm^{-1} when concentration is in mole per liter constant is called molar absorptivity and has the symbol ε so the equation becomes as:

$$A = \varepsilon bc \text{ units of } \varepsilon \text{ are mol}^{-1} cm^{-1}$$

Limitations to Beer's Law

Deviations from the direct proportionality between the measured absorbance and concentration when b is constant are encountered (Skoog, 2004).

Generally three types of deviation are:
1. Real limitation of the law
2. Chemical deviation
3. Instrumental deviation

Real limitation of the Beer's law

Beer's law successfully described absorption behavior of low concentration media but at high concentration usually > 0.01 m the average distance between the molecule responsible for the absorption is diminished to the point where each molecule effect the charge distribution of its neighbors. This interaction in turn, can alter the ability of the molecule to absorb a given wavelength of radiation, while the effect of molecular interaction is ordinary not significant at concentration below 0.01 m. Deviations also arise because of ε which is dependent upon the refractive index of medium.

Chemical deviation

Apparent deviation from Beer's law arises when an analyte dissociates, associate or reacts with a solvent.

Instrumental deviation

- Polychromatic radiation: strict adherence to Beer's law is observed only with true monochromatic radiation

- In the presence of stray radiation often differs greatly in wavelength from that of the principle and in addition may not have pass through the sample.

Absorbance then observed as:

$$A' = \log p_0 + p_s/p + p_s$$

where

p_s is power of non absorbed stray radiation

p_0 is power of incident light

p is power of transmitted light

Instrument components: UV-Visible Spectrophotometer is made up of

1. *Source:* For the purpose of molecular absorption measurements, a continuum source is required whose power does not change sharply over a considerable range of wavelengths. E.g., Deuterium and hydrogen lamps, tungsten filament lamps, xenon arc lamps.

2. *Wavelength selector:* Although prisms can be used as monochromators, most instruments use diffraction gratings. Light shining on the closely spaced grooves of a diffraction grating at an angle is separated into different wavelengths in a consistent manner.

3. ***Sample container:*** Most samples studied using visible and ultraviolet spectroscopy is liquid. The sample must therefore be placed in a transparent container to allow measurement. These containers are called cuvettes. They should be constructed of a material that passes radiation in the spectral region of interest. Quartz and fused silica is required for work in the ultraviolet region (below 350 nm) and they are also transparent in the visible region.

4. ***Detector:*** The most commonly used detector is a **photomultiplier tube** (PMT). An incoming photon hits a thin metal film inside a vacuum tube. The metal film is maintained at a large negative potential and emits electrons. These collide with a series of dynodes maintained at progressively lower potentials; each dynode emits several electrons in response to each incoming electron, resulting in a large amplification of the signal.

Types of instruments

Single beam spectrophotometer: A single beam spectrophotometer is comprised of a light source, a monochromator, a sample holder and a detector (Figure 19.2). An ideal instrument has a light source that emits with equal intensity at all wavelengths, a monochromator that is equally efficient in splitting light into narrow groups of wavelength for all wavelengths and a detector that is sensitive and responds equally to all wavelengths.

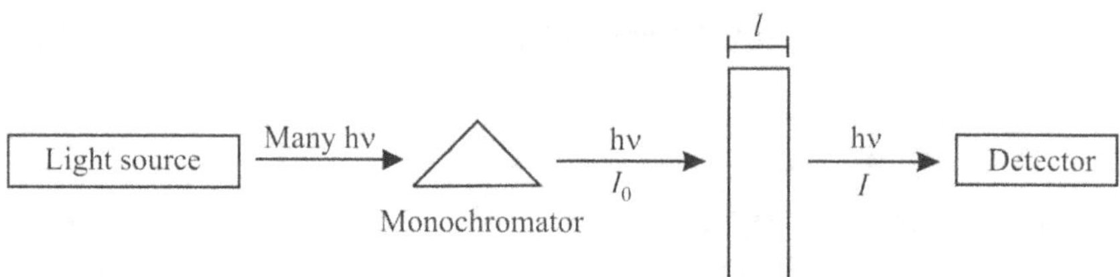

Fig. 19.2 Instrument design for single beam spectrophotometer.

Double beam spectrophotometer: Modern spectrophotometers are based on double-beam design. Figure 19.3 illustrates a double beam instrument in which two beams are formed by a rotating sector mirror. The entire beam first passes through the reference cell and then through the sample cell. The pulses of radiation are recombined by another sector mirror which reflects one pulse and transmits other to the detector.

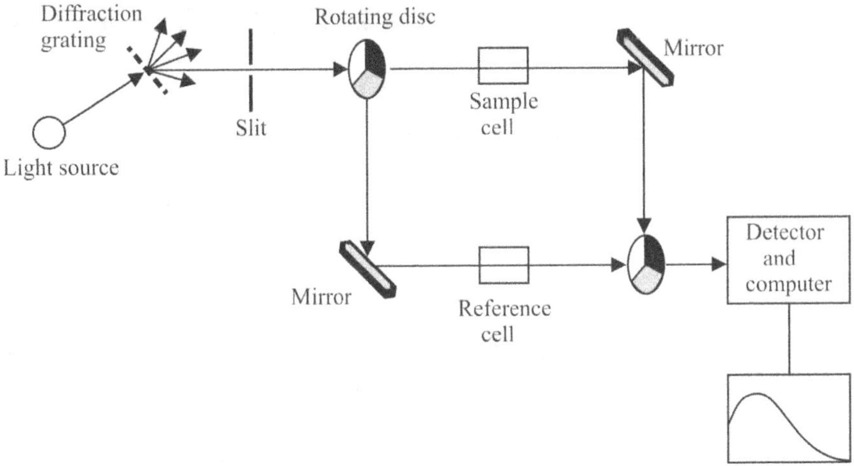

Fig. 19.3 Instrument design for double beam spectrophotometer.

Experiment 19.1

To Verify Beer-Lambert's Law

Theory

Absorption spectroscopy can be used to quantify the absorbing species present in the sample. The greater the quantity of absorbing species present, the greater will be the extent to which the incident light will be absorbed. When a beam of monochromatic light falls on a substance, a part of it is absorbed and the rest is transmitted. The intensity of the transmitted light is decreased. According to Lambert's law, decrease in intensity ($-dI$) is proportional to the thickness of the medium (dl) and intensity of incident light (I). Beer extended this law towards solutions (and gases). In such cases decrease in intensity is also proportional to molar concentration (C).

So, $- dI = K.\ I.\ dl.\ C$ (K is a constant)

Beer-Lambert's law states that for a solution, the absorbance of the sample (A) is given by:

$$A = \log (I_0 / I) = \varepsilon\, C\, l = O.\ D.$$

where, I_0 is the intensity of the incident light,

I is the intensity of the transmitted light,

ε is the molar absorptivity (characteristic of the absorbing species),

C is the molar concentration of the absorbing species in the sample,

l is the distance that the incident radiation travels through the sample.

$\log (I_0 / I)$ = Optical density or Absorbance

Since ε depends on wave length of the light and nature of the substance so for a given substance at a given frequency and in a given photochemical cell (l = constant), O.D. = constant $\times$ C. Hence, a plot of O.D. Vs C will be a straight line through origin. This is Beer's law. Absorbance has no units. If 'l' is expressed in cm and 'C' in mol dm^{-3}, then 'ε' has the units of $mol^{-1}dm^{3}\ cm^{-1}$. A linear plot of absorbance versus concentration would verify the Beer-Lambert's Law.

Chemicals required

1. Potassium permanganate stock solution (0.005M).

2. Distilled water.

Procedure

Verification of Beer-Lambert's Law

1. A stock solution of 0.005M is to be prepared for 100 mL. From this solution, 20 mL is pipetted out into a 100 mL standard flask and make up to the mark with distilled water. This is the standard solution of 0.001M $KMnO_4$ solution.

2. Record the visible spectrum of this solution (0.001M $KMnO_4$) in the wavelength range of 350 nm to 800 nm (at the intervals of 10 nm to get maximum wavelength i.e., λ_{max}). Note your results in Table 19.1.

3. A plot of Absorbance (A) vs Wave length (nm) gives λ_{max}.

4. Prepare 10 mL solutions of the following proportions of $KMnO_4$ solution given in the Table 19.2, from the standard solution.

5. Measure the absorbance (A) at λmax for each of the solutions prepared in Step 4 and for the unknown solution of $KMnO_4$ also. Note your results in Table 19.2.

6. Plot a graph between Absorbance (y-axis) vs Concentration (x-axis).

Table 19.1 Determination of λ_{max} for 0.001M $KMnO_4$.

S. No.	Wavelength, λ (nm)	Absorbance (A)

Table 19.2 Absorbance of $KMnO_4$ solutions at λ_{max} (................nm).

S. No.	Volume of 0.001 M KMnO$_4$ (mL)	Volume of water (mL)	Concentration of KMnO$_4$ (M)	Absorbance
1	10.0	0.0		
2	7.5	2.5		
3	5.0	5.0		
4	2.5	7.5		
5	1.0	9.0		
6	X	Y		

Observation and Calculations

Concentration of the unknown solution is read out from the calibration curve and the nature of the calibration curve is to be determined.

Experiment 19.2

Determination of Salicylic Acid in Synthesized Aspirin by UV-Spectrophotometric Method

Theory

The purity of the synthesized aspirin can be tested by addition of ferric to a suspension of the product. Phenols (such as salicylic acid) react with ferric chloride to form colored complex. The complex formed between ferric ion and salicylic acid is blue, which allow its visual detection. Obviously, the intensity of the observed color is proportional to the complex concentration. Complex concentration can be determined by Spectrophotometric measurement of the absorbance of the complex in the visible region (540 nm). The $FeCl_3$ solution is added to a sample of aspirin unpurified with salicylic acid to form complex. Absorbance of the solution is determined. The concentration of the complex and therefore the purity of the aspirin, will be calculated from the standard curve.

Chemicals required

1. 5% $FeCl_3$ (aq).

2. 0.2M salicylic acid (Mol. Wt. = 138) in ethanol.

Procedure

1. Qualitative determination of the residual salicylic acid

(i)   The purity of the synthesized aspirin can be tested by addition of Fe^{+3} to a suspension of the product.

(ii) Prepare a tube with a small amount (a few crystals) of aspirin.

(iii) Add water (2 mL) and 1 mL of 0.1% aqueous solution of $FeCl_3$.

(iv) The color development is considered a positive test and is an indication of the presence of salicylic acid.

2. Quantitative determination of the residual salicylic acid by spectrophotometry

(i) **Preparation of the calibration curve:** A series of standard complex solutions will be prepared and their absorbance measured at 540 nm in a spectrophotometer. Concentration of solutions must be ranged between 1×10^{-4} and 8×10^{-4} M.

   (a) Prepare five 50 mL volumetric flasks.

   (b) In each one, put the volume (mL) of solutions indicated in the table below. Add water up to the mark.

   (c) Add distilled water to fill the flask up to 50 mL.

   (d) Measure the absorbance of the solutions at wavelength 540 nm.

   (e) Plot the calibration curve: Absorbance vs. concentration (M)

Flask number	Volume of 0.2M salicylic acid (mL)	Volume of 5% $FeCl_3$ (mL)	Concentration of solution (mol/L)
1	0.5	0.1	1×10^{-4}
2	1.0	0.2	2×10^{-4}
3	2.0	0.4	4×10^{-4}
4	3.0	0.6	6×10^{-4}
5	4.0	0.8	8×10^{-4}

(ii) **Preparation of the aspirin sample**

   (a) Place 0.2 g of aspirin into a 50 mL flask.

   (b) Add ethanol (5 mL approximately) to dissolve it.

   (c) Add a 1 mL solution of $FeCl_3$, and fill flask up to mark (if a precipitate appears, add a little more ethanol and dilute after that to 50 mL).

   (d) The observed color must be included in the calibration scale.

   (e) If the observed color is too intense, dilute the solution.

(iii) Determination of salicylic acid concentration in aspirin sample

    (a) Measure the absorbance of the sample solution by means of the spectrophotometer.

    (b) Use the calibration curve to calculate the concentration of the complexed salicylic acid (C) in the solution.

Observation and Calculations

% Salicylic acid in aspirin

$$\text{salicylic acid } \% = \frac{C \times 50 \times 10^{-3} \times 138}{0.2}$$

Experiment 19.3

Determination of Paracetamol Content in Tablet by UV-Spectrophotometric Method

Theory

Paracetamol is a widely used over-the-counter analgesic and antipyretic. It is commonly used for fever, headache and other minor aches and pain, and is a major ingredient in numerous cold and flu remedies. In combination with other non-steroidal anti-inflammatory drugs (NSAIDs) or opioid analgesics, paracetamol is used also in the management of more severe pain.

It shows three λ_{max} at 242, 243 and 257 nm in neutral, acidic and alkaline medium respectively. The present experiment is an estimation of paracetamol, in alkaline media. Paracetamol shows maximum absorption at 257 nm due to presence of phenyl ring in alkaline medium. The absorbance of different dilution of paracetamol is taken at this wavelength to make the calibration curve. The absorbance of unknown sample is taken and with the help of calibration curve, the concentration is read out.

Chemical equation

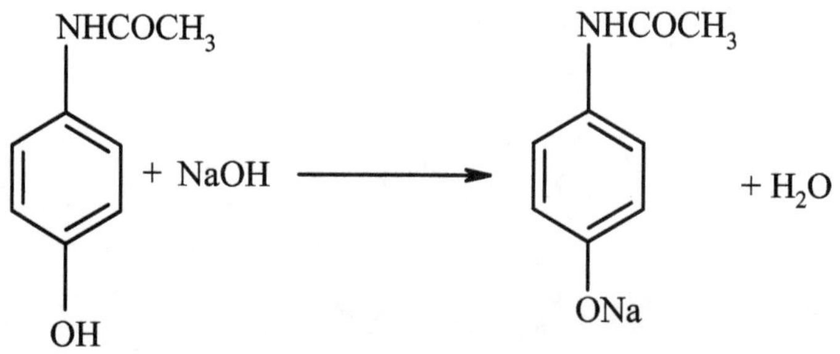

$$NHCOCH_3\text{-}C_6H_4\text{-}OH + NaOH \longrightarrow NHCOCH_3\text{-}C_6H_4\text{-}ONa + H_2O$$

Paracetamol + NaOH ⟶ Sodium salt of paracetamol + H₂O

Chemicals required

1. Paracetamol.

2. Sodium hydroxide (NaOH).

Procedure

(i) Accurately weigh 100 mg of paracetamol reference substance and transfer it into a 100 mL volumetric flask.

(ii) Dissolve it with 50 mL of 0.01M NaOH solution.

(iii) Dilute to volume with water and mix well.

(iv) Separately transfer accurately 0.1 to 1 mL of this solution into 10 different 10 mL volumetric flask and dilute with 0.1M NaOH solution to the mark making the concentration range from 0.32-1.92 mg/mL.

(v) Measure the absorbance of the each solution at 257 nm.

(vi) Weigh accurately and powder finely 10 tablets, weigh accurately a portion of the powder (equivalent to about 100 mg of paracetamol) into 100 mL volumetric flask, add 50 ml of 0.1M NaOH solution, mix for 15 minutes.

(vii) Filter if necessary.

(viii) Make up the volume with 0.1M NaOH solution.

(ix) Transfer 0.5 mL of this solution and dilute to 10 mL in volumetric flask.

Observation and Calculations

1. Plot a calibration curve by plotting a graph between absorbance of different standard dilution and their concentration.

2. Read out a concentration of unknown from calibration curve.

3. Multiply the concentration with dilution factor to find out the initial concentration.

Experiment 19.4

Determination of Amoxycillin Content in Capsule by UV- Spectrophotometric Method

Theory

Amoxycillin is a moderate spectrum, Beta-lactam antibiotic used to treat bacterial infections caused by susceptible microorganism. The capsule contains 250 or 500 mg of $C_{16}H_{19}N_3O_5S$, calculated with reference to anhydrous base. Its structure is:

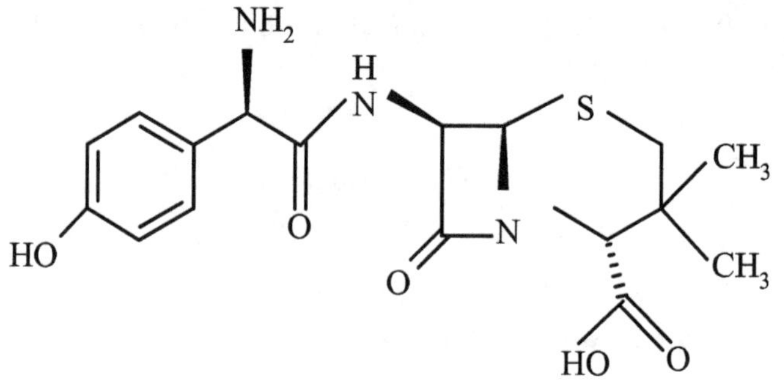

Chemicals required

(i)   Amoxycillin reference substance.

(ii)   *p*-Dimethylaminobenzaldehyde. Dissolve 0.4 g of *p*-Dimethyl-aminobenzaldehyde in 10 mL of alcohol. Add to it 2 mL of conc. Sulfuric acid solution. Make up the volume to 50 mL with water.

(iii) Alcohol.

Procedure

1. Preparation of standard amoxicillin solution:

    (i)   Weigh accurately about 150 mg of amoxicillin and transfer it to a volumetric flask.

    (ii) Dissolve it in sufficient distilled water and make up the volume up to 100 mL volumetric flask to form the stock solution of concentration 1.5 mg/mL of amoxicillin.

    (iii) From this solution, take 0.1 to 10 mL of solution in 10 different flask and make up the volume to 10 mL.

    (iv) From above standard solution, pipette out 2 mL and add 4 mL of p-Dimethylaminobenzaldehyde.

    (v) Heat for 1 hr on a water bath.

    (vi) Cool down and make up the volume to 10 mL with distilled water in volumetric flask.

2. Preparation of test sample solution:

    (i)   Weigh accurately 20 capsules and find out the average weight of capsule.

    (ii) Weigh accurately powder equivalent to 150 mg of amoxicillin and transfer it to a volumetric flask.

    (iii) Dissolve in sufficient distilled water and make up the volume to 100 mL.

    (iv) Take 1 mL of this solution and dilute up to 10 mL with distilled water in volumetric flask.

    (v) Pipette out 2 mL of amoxicillin, add 4 mL of p-Dimethyl-aminobenzaldehyde and heat on water bath for 1 hr. Cool down and make up the volume to 10 mL.

    (vi) Measure the absorbance of each standard and test sample at 410 nm.

Observation and Calculations

Average weight of capsule: W_1 g.

Average weight of capsule powder equivalent to 150 mg of amoxicillin: W_2 g.

Plot a calibration curve by plotting a graph between concentrations of solution (μg) vs absorbance. Read out the concentration of test solution from the calibration curve.

Suppose, it is 20 μg

The amount of amoxicillin in the sample = $20 \times 100 \times 10 \times 5$

$$= 100,000 \ \mu g = 100 \ mg$$

Where $100 \times 10 \times 5$ is the dilution factor

W_2 g test sample contain = 100 mg of amoxicillin

Experiment 19.5

Determination of Eflornithine Hydrochloride in Parenteral Formulation by UV-Spectro-photometric Method

Theory

Eflornithine hydrochloride (DL-alpha-Difluoromethylornithine; DFMO) has the IUPAC name 2,5-diamino-2-(difluoromethyl) pentanoic acid. Anhydrous eflornithine hydrochloride has molecular formula $C_6H_{12}F_2N_2O_2.HCl$ and a molecular weight of 218.65. Eflornithine is a specific, irreversible inhibitor of the enzyme ornithine decarboxylase, one of the key enzymes in the polyamine biosynthetic pathway. The drug was originally developed for use in cancer and is in phase III clinical trials for its use in preventing recurrence of superficial bladder cancer. It has been used as antiprotozoal agent in the treatment of meningoencephalic stage of trypanosomiasis caused by *Trypanosoma brucei gambienze* (African trypanosomiasis). It is now licensed for use in sleeping sickness in FDA, US, Europe and twelve African countries.

Chemicals required

1. Eflornithine hydrochloride

2. Ethanol

Procedure

1. Preparation of stock solution of reference substance

(i) Prepare a stock solution of 1.0 mg/mL is dissolving 100 mg of DFMO in a 100 mL of ethanol.

(ii) Prepare working standard solution of DFMO of 100 µg/mL was by appropriate dilution of the stock solution with ethanol.

(iii) Pipette out 2.0 mL aliquot of standard DFMO solution of 10 µg/mL into a 10 mL volumetric flask.

(iv) The volume is made up to 10 mL with ethanol and solution and then scanned in the range of 200 to 400 nm against the reagent blank.

(v) The absorbance values are recorded and absorption maxima of (DFMO) 20 µg/mLs should be 283 nm.

2. Preparation of sample solution

(i) Use twenty vials of Eflornithine hydrochloride.

(ii) The sample vial containing 200 mg/mL.

(iii) Pipette out 1 mL and dilute to 100 mL with ethanol.

(iv) Further dilute the solution with ethanol to get the final concentration of 100 µg/mL.

(v) Dilute appropriately by using ethanol.

(vi) Pipette out aliquots of 0.4 mL, 0.8 mL, 1.2 mL, 1.6 mL, 2.0 mL, 2.4 mL, 2.8 mL and 3.2 mL of 100 µg/mL solution of DFMO into each of 10 mL volumetric flasks.

(vii) Make up the volume up to 10 mL with ethanol and measure the absorbance of solution w 283 nm against ethanol as blank.

Observation and Calculations

$$\text{Absorbance} = \varepsilon bc$$

where, ε = slope in a plot of Absorbance versus concentration

$c = \Delta$ Absorbance/ Δ concentration

$b = 1$ cm

Experiment 19.6

Determination of Albendazole in Suspension Forms by UV-Spectrophotometric Method

Theory

Albendazole is a broad spectrum anthelmintic. It is used for the treatment of Threadworm, Hookworm and Tapeworm. Chemically, Albendazole is Methyl 5-propylthio-1H-benzimidazol-2-yl carbamate.

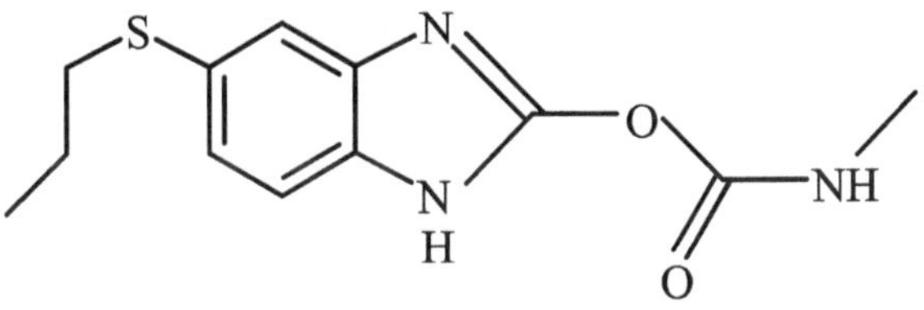

Albendazole

Chemicals required

1. Albendazole

2. Distilled water

Procedure

1. **Preparation of Albendazole stock solution**

   (i) Prepare standard stock solution by dissolving 50 mg of standard Albendazole in 100 mL of methanolic glacial acetic acid to get concentration of 500 µg/mL.

2. Procedure for calibration curve

(i) Further dilute the aliquots of stock solution with methanolic glacial acetic acid to get working solution of 2.5, 5.0, 7.5, 10.0, 12.5, 15.0, 17.5, 20.0 and 22.5 µg/mL.

(ii) Subsequently, the prepared standards are measured after standing for 5 min at λ_{max} in each case against a solvent blank similarly prepared.

(iii) Plot the calibration curve of absorbance against the concentration of the drug.

3. Procedure for pharmaceutical preparation

(i) Accurately weigh a suspension equivalent to 100 mg of albendazole and transfer to 100 ml volumetric flask and dissolve in 20 mL methanolic glacial acetic acid.

(ii) Shake the solution for 20 min.

(iii) Further dilute the resulting solution to 100 mL with methanolic acetic acid and filter through Whatman filter paper no 41.

(iv) Pipette out 1 mL of the above solution into 100 mL volumetric flask and make up to the mark.

(v) Measure the absorbance against the blank at 235 nm.

(vi) Calculate the amount of drug from the calibration curve.

Observation and Calculations

1. Plot a calibration curve by plotting a graph between absorbance of different standard dilution and their concentration.

2. Read out a concentration of unknown from calibration curve (Figure 19.4).

3. Multiply the concentration with dilution factor to find out the initial concentration.

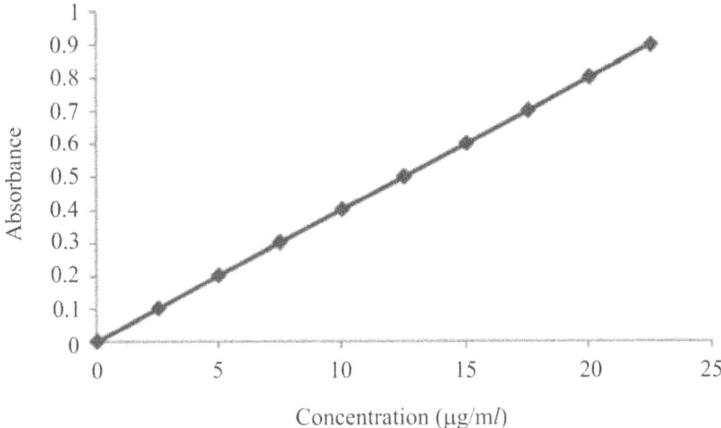

Fig. 19.4 Calibration curve of albendazole at 235 nm.

Experiment 19.7

Determination of Ranitidine in Tablet Dosage Form Spectrophotometrically

Theory

Ranitidine is a histamine H_2-receptor antagonist that inhibits stomach acid production. It is commonly used in treatment of peptic ulcer disease and gastro-esophageal reflux disease. Chemically it is *N*-(2-[(5-[(di-methylamino)methyl]furan-2-yl)methylthio]ethyl)-*N'*-methyl-2-nitroethene-1,1-diamine.

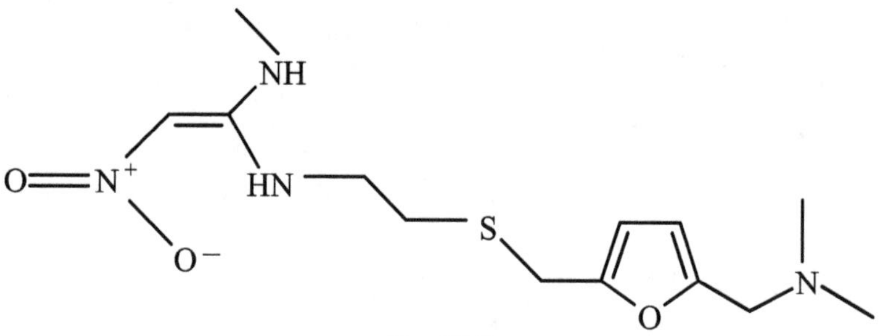

Ranitidine

Chemicals required

1. Ranitidine HCl (reference standard).
2. Distilled water.

Procedure

1. Preparation of standard Ranitidine HCl solution

(i)   Weigh accurately 100 mg of ranitidine HCl.

(ii) Dissolve in sufficient distilled water and make up the volume to 100 mL in volumetric flask.

(iii) Pipette out 2 mL of this solution in 100 mL volume flask and make up the volume.

(iv) Measure the absorbance of above solution at 313 nm (λ_{max} of ranitidine).

2. Preparation of unknown Ranitidine HCl solution

(i) Weigh accurately 20 tablets and calculate their average weight.

(ii) Powder the tablets and weigh accurately the powder equivalent to 100 mg of ranitidine HCl.

(iii) Transfer it to 100 mL volumetric flask, dissolve in sufficient distilled water and make up the volume.

(iv) Pipette out 2 ml of the above solution, transfer it to a 100 mL volumetric flask and make up the volume with distilled water.

(v) Measure the absorbance of above solution at 313 nm (λ_{max} of ranitidine).

Observation and Calculations

Average weight of tablet = W_1 g

Weight of powder equivalent to 100 mg of rantidine HCl = W_2 g

Weight of standard ranitidine HCl = W_3 g

Absorbance of standard ranitidine HCl = A_1

Absorbance of test ranitidine HCl = A_2

$$\text{The content of Ranitidine in tablet} = \frac{A_2 \times W_3 \times 314.37 \times 99}{A_1 \times W_2 \times 350.87 \times 100} \times W_1$$

314.37 and 350.87 are the molecular weights of Ranitidine base and Ranitidine HCl respectively.

Experiment 19.8

Simultaneous Estimation of Cefixime and Ofloxacin in Tablet Dosage Form Spectrophotometrically

Theory

Cefixime, a third generation cephalosporin antibiotic, chemically is (6*R*,7*R*)-7-{[2-(2-amino-1,3-thiazol-4-yl)-2-(carboxymethoxyimino)acetyl] amino}-3-ethenyl-8-oxo-5-thia-1-azabicyclo[4.2.0]oct-2-ene-2-carboxylic acid. The Cephalosporins are a class of β-lactam antibiotics originally derived from *Acremonium*, which was previously known as "Cephalosporium".

Cefixime

Ofloxacin is a synthetic chemotherapeutic antibiotic of the fluoroquinolone drug class considered to be a second-generation fluoroquinolone (Nelson, 2007; Kawahara, 1998). Chemically it is (RS)-7-fluoro-2-methyl-6-(4-methylpiperazin-1-yl)-10-oxo-4-oxa-1-azatricyclo [7.3.1.05,13]trideca-5(13),6,8,11-tetraene-11-carboxylic acid.

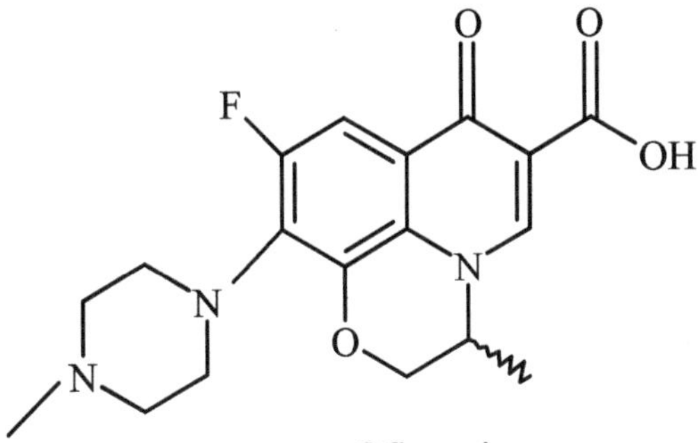

Ofloxacin

Chemicals required:

1. Ofloxacin - 200 mg

2. Cefixime trihydrate - 200 mg

3. Methanol

Procedure

1. **Preparation of stock solution and determination of absorption maxima**

   (i) Weigh 20 mg each of Cefixime and Ofloxacin separately and then dissolve in methanol and then make the volume up to 50 ml with methanol to give 400 µg/mL of each solution and use it for further analysis.

   (ii) Dilute the stock solution to 10 µg/mL of Cefixime and 10 µg/ml of Ofloxacin respectively and then scan separately in the range of 200-400 nm to determine the wavelength of maximum absorption of both the drugs.

   (iii) Cefixime has maximum absorption at 288.7 nm and Ofloxacin at 295.3 nm.

2. **Estimation of sample**

   (i) Two wavelengths selected for the method are 288.7 nm (λ_1) and 295.3 nm (λ_2) that are absorption maximas of Cefixime and Ofloxacin respectively.

   (ii) Further dilute the stock solution of the samples was methanol separately to get standard solutions of concentrations 5, 10, 15 µg/mL.

(iii) Measure the absorbance of these solutions at selected wavelengths and determine the absorptivity of these as a mean of three independent determinations.

3. **Determination of Linearity Range**

(i) The linearity of this method can be evaluated by linear regression analysis and calculated by least square method. The drug shows linearity in the concentration range of 2-34 µg/ml for Cefixime and 2-20 µg/ml for Ofloxacin.

(ii) Prepare the standard dilutions using the required volume from the stock solution and make the required volume with methanol to yield the concentrations.

(iii) Measure the absorbance of the resulting solutions and plot the calibration curve between absorbance and concentration of the drug.

4. **Limit of detection and quantification**

(i) Limit of detection (LOD) is the minimum concentration of the analyte in the sample which can be analyzed by the instrument.

(ii) Limit of quantification (LOQ) is the minimum concentration of the analyte that can be reliably quantified.

(iii) These parameters were calculated for the proposed methods based on the standard deviation (SD) of the y-intercept and the slope (m) of the calibration curves.

Observation and Calculations

1. **Concentration of the drug in the samples can be obtained using the following equations**

$$C_x = \frac{A_1 ay_2 - A_2 ay_1}{ax_1 ay_2 - ax_2 ay_1}$$

$$C_y = \frac{A_1 ax_2 - A_2 ax_1}{ay_1 ax_2 - ay_2 ax_1}$$

where A_1 and A_2 are absorbance of mixture at 288.7 and 295.3 nm respectively, ax_1 and ax_2 are the absorptivities of Cefixime at λ_1 and λ_2 respectively and ay_1, ay_2 are the absorptivities of Ofloxacin at λ_1 and λ_2 respectively. C_x and C_y are the concentrations of Cefixime and Ofloxacin in g/L respectively.

2. Determination of Linearity Range

Linearity of the calibration curve is measured from regression equation:

$$y = mx + c$$

where m = Slope or Gradient

         b = the Y Intercept

3. Limit of detection and quantification

$$LOD = 3.3 \ (SD/m)$$

$$LOQ = 10 \ (SD/m)$$

CHAPTER 20

Infrared Spectrophotometry

Infrared Spectrophotometry

The region in the electromagnetic radiation spectrum extending from 0.8 to 200 μ is known as infrared. This can be further split into three parts namely:

    (a) 0.8 to 2.5 μ or 12500 to 4000 cm^{-1} (near IR)

    (b) 2.5 μ to 15 μ or 4000 to 667 cm^{-1} (ordinary IR) and

    (c) 15 to 200 μ or 667 to 50 cm^{-1} (far IR).

Most of our attention will be focused on the region between 0.8 to 50 μ because this can be explored with the aid of commercial instruments and also where in the spectra arise mainly from the stretching and bending movements of atoms within molecules. The infrared spectra are used for the identification and study of molecular structure of compounds.

Theory

Infrared radiations of frequencies less than 100 cm^{-1} is absorbed and converted by an organic molecule into energy of molecular rotation. This absorption is quantized and thus molecular rotation spectrum consists of discrete lines. Infrared radiations of frequencies between 10,000-100 cm^{-1} is absorbed and converted by an organic molecule into energy of molecular vibration. This absorption is quantized and vibrational spectrum appears in the form of bands rather than discrete lines because a single vibrational energy change comprises of a set of rotational energy changes.

There are two kinds of fundamental vibrations:

(a) *Stretching:* In these vibrations, distance between the two atoms increases or decreases, but atoms remain in the same bond axis. The stretching is of two types (a) symmetrical stretching (b) asymmetrical stretching. For example, in a three-atom system like

H-C-H the symmetrical stretching will have two hydrogen atoms move towards and away from the central atom of carbon in unison, altering the inter-atomic distance without change in the valence angle.

In asymmetrical stretching, one hydrogen atom will approach the carbon while the other will move away from carbon.

(b) *Bending:* In these vibrations, the position of the atom changes relative to original bond axis. There are four types of bending vibrations: namely,

(a) *Wagging*: the structural unit swings back and forth in the plane of the molecule (in plane bending).

(b) *Rocking*: the structural unit swings back and forth out of the plane of the molecule (out of plane bending).

(c) *Twisting*: the structural unit rotates about the bond which joins it to the rest of the molecule.

(d) *Scissoring*: the two atoms connected to a central atom move towards and away from each other with deformation of valence angle.

The two most important requirements for a substance to absorb infrared radiation are:

(a) That the natural frequency of vibration of the molecule is same as the frequency of vibration and

(b) That the vibration so produced brings about a change in the dipole moment of the molecule.

The positions of the centers of gravity of the positive and negative electrical charges between two dissimilar atoms in a molecule will determine its dipole moment. If the values of the dipole moment in the extreme positions differ, a periodically changing electrical field will be set around the molecule. As a consequence, absorption of radiant energy at the vibrating frequencies will take place. In this manner a resonance condition will be established. But diatomic molecules like H_2, N_2, O_2 and ethylene do not absorb any infrared radiation. They are homopolar molecules and do not produce a dipole moment due to their symmetry. In a molecule like CO_2, no dipole moment is created in the symmetrical stretching vibration because the centers of gravity coincide in every vibrational positional position. But in the case of the asymmetrical stretching vibrations, the centers of gravity of the charges do not coincide. A dipole moment is produced and absorption characteristic of this mode is absorbed in the infrared spectrum.

The intensity of infrared absorption band is proportional to the square of the rate of change of dipole moment with respect to the displacement of the atoms. Thus when the magnitude of change in dipole moment is small, a weak absorption band will be obtained, e.g., $C\equiv N$ group. If the change in dipole moment is very large, a strong absorption band will be obtained, e.g., $C=O$ group.

Radiation sources

The light from the source falls on a concave spherical mirror which condenses the radiation into an image of the source and then fills the entrance slit of the monochromator. The common sources of infrared are:

(a) *Nernst glower:* It is made up of a mixture of zirconium and yttrium oxides. It is heated to a temperature of 1500-2000 °C and furnish maximum radiation of about 7100 cm^{-1}.

(b) *Globar:* It consists of a rod of silicon carbide and is heated up to 1300-1700 °C furnishing maximum radiation of about 5200 cm^{-1}.

(c) *Nichrome wire:* Coils of nichrome wire are also used as a source in infrared spectrophotometer. These coils are heated up to 800-900 °C.

Monochromators

A monochromator is a device for isolating narrow wavelength regions from a source of heterogeneous light. It consists of a dispersing element which may be a prism or a grating together with two narrow slits to serve as entrance and exit parts for the radiation. The entrance slit allows a narrow beam to fall on the dispersing device which deflects the beam through an angle depending on the wavelength. The beam thus fans out and is focused into the exit slit which then allows a narrow band of wavelength to pass through into the detector section. The sample and reference are placed at or near a focus of the beam just before the entrance slit to the monochromator. A collimating mirror which is an off-axis section of a large parabolic mirror is placed in front of the entrance slit to make the light parallel and sent to the dispersing device.

Detectors

The detectors suitable for infrared spectroscopy are of two types:

(a) *Thermal detectors:* A thermal detector is based on the absorption of energy of a large number of incident photons to produce a response through their heating effects. Thermal detectors can be used over a wider range of wavelength and do not need cooling.

(b) ***Photon detectors:*** A photon detector is a semiconductor device in which an electron absorbs the energy of a single quantum of infrared radiation and is promoted from valence band to the conduction band producing electrical conductivity. Photon detectors are fast and more sensitive than thermal detector, but are restricted in wavelength and need cooling.

Sample handling

The techniques for analyzing the samples by IR spectroscopy differ for solid, liquid and gaseous materials. For gaseous samples, gas cells equipped with mirrors to allow the radiation to pass through are commercially available. However, sample preparation requires prior removal of water vapor. For solids or powders, a common way of examining them is convert them into a mull or thick slurry. The powdered sample is mixed (10-15 mg) with a greasy, liquid medium (a few drops) like paraffin oil, nujol, hexachlorobutadiene, perfluorokerose etc., and form a paste. The suspension thus prepared is then sandwiched between two NaCl plates and mounted on a demountable cell holder. This technique may give difficulties due to scattering of radiation. Therefore the liquid medium should possess approximately same refractive index to reduce energy losses.

Another technique adopted for solid samples is by converting them into a disk or pallet of potassium bromide. A weighed portion of powdered sample (1.0 mg) is thoroughly mixed in a small ball mill with a weighed quantity of purified and desiccated KBr powder (200 mg). The mixture is placed in an evacuable die and subjected to a pressure of 10-15 Torr. A highly transparent disk or a pallet is produced which is then placed in a pallet holder and IR scanned. The disk is about 1 cm in diameter and about 0.5 mm thick.

Samples which are liquid at room temperature are generally examined in their pure form. The procedure is called thin film technique or neat form. A thin layer of the sample is sandwiched between two salt plates and then fixed into a demountable cell holder provided with gaskets. The sample thickness should be such that the transmittance lies between 15 to 70%. Liquid samples with high viscosity cannot be analyzed as such and therefore need to be dissolved in suitable solvents. The solvents should be non-absorbing in the region of interest. Carbon tetrachloride is satisfactory but absorbs between 800-740 cm^{-1} (12.5-13.5 μ), carbon disulphide absorbs at 2222 cm^{-1} (4.5 μ) and 1540 cm^{-1} (6.5 μ). Solvents chosen should be free from moisture and hydrogen bonding effects. Chloroform, cyclohexane and similar solvents can also be used in a restricted manner.

The absorption cells available for liquid samples are called sealed cells or preassembled cells. It consists of a pair of salt plates separated by a shim or gasket made of a metal or Teflon and held together like sandwich between two metals clamps. Two holes are drilled through the metal frame and to the salt plates for filling and emptying. The cell can be filled and rinsed with the help of a hypodermic syringe. Such cells are demountable type provided with fittings.

Table 20.1 Principal absorption bands of selected functional groups.

Functional group	Wavenumber (cm^{-1})	Intensity
C–H Stretching		
Alkanes	2850-3300	
Alkenes	(3.51-3.03 μ) region.	m-s
Alkynes	C≡C–H stretching characteristically	s
Aromatic hydrocarbons	located near 3300	
Aldehyde C–H	Two bands 2800-2900 cm^{-1} and 2700-2780 cm^{-1}	w
C–H bending		
Alkanes	1340-1480	m – s
Alkenes	1300-1420	s
	800-1000	s
Alkynes	630	s
Aromatic	700-900	v
C–C double bond triple bond stretching		
Alkenes	1620-1680	w-m
Alkynes	2100-2300	w-m
Carbonyl C=O stretching		
Aldehydes		
Saturated aliphatic	1720 -1740	s
α,β – unsaturated aliphatic	1680-1705	s
Aryl	1680-1715	s
Ketones		
Saturated aliphatic	1705-1750	s
α,β – unsaturated aliphatic	1660-1685	s
Aryl	1680-1700	s

Table 20.1 *Contd...*

Functional group	Wavenumber (cm^{-1})	Intensity
Esters		
Saturated	1735-1750	s
α, β – unsaturated aliphatic	1715-1730	s
Aryl	1715-1730	s
Saturated γ-lactones	1760-1780	s
Saturated β-lactones	~ 1820	s
α, β – unsaturated γ-lactones	1740-1760	s
γ, β – unsaturated γ-lactones	1800	s
Ketoesters	~1650	s
Carboxylic acids		
Saturated	1700-1725	s
α, β – unsaturated aliphatic	1690-1715	s
Aryl	1680-1700	s
Caboxylate ion	1550-1610	s
	1300-1400	s
Amides		
Solid or concentrated solution	1630-1680	s
Dilute solution	1670-1700	s
Lactams	1680-1780	s
Ureas	1660-1730	s
Imides	1670-1700	s
	1700-1730	s
Alcohols and phenols (O-H stretching)		
Free OH	3590-3650	v
Hydrogen-bonded OH	3450-3650	v
N-H stretching		
1°	~3400	m
2°	~3500	m
Amine salts	3000-3150	m
N-H bending in 1° and 2° salts	1550-1650	m^{-s}
	1570-1600	s
C-N stretching		
Aliphatic	1000-1200	w
	1400	w
Aromatic	1250-1350	s

Table 20.1 *Contd...*

Functional group	Wavenumber (cm^{-1})	Intensity
Nitrites and isocyanides (C≡N stretching)		
Nitriles	2220-2280	m
Isocyanides	2050-2220	m
Nitro compounds (N-O stretching)		
Aromatic, asymmetric	1500-1570	s
Aromatic, symmetric	1300-1370	s
Aliphatic, asymmetric	1500-1570	s
Aliphatic, symmetric	1370-1380	s
Halogen compounds		
C-Cl stretching	600-800	s
C-Br stretching	500-650	s
C-I stretching	500-600	s
Sulphur compounds		
S-H stretching	2550-2600	w
Thiocarbonyl compounds; C=S stretching	1050-1200	
S=O stretching	1140-1180	s
	1300-1350	s

Intensity: s, strong; m, medium; w, weak; v, variable

Experiment 20.1

To Interpret IR Spectra of Paracetamol

Theory

Paracetamol, chemically named N-acetyl-p-aminophenol is a analgesic and a anti-pyretic. Paracetamol is used to treat many conditions such as headache, muscle aches, arthritis, backache, toothaches, colds, and fevers. It relieves pain in mild arthritis but has no effect on the underlying inflammation and swelling of the joint.

Spectra of Paracetamol

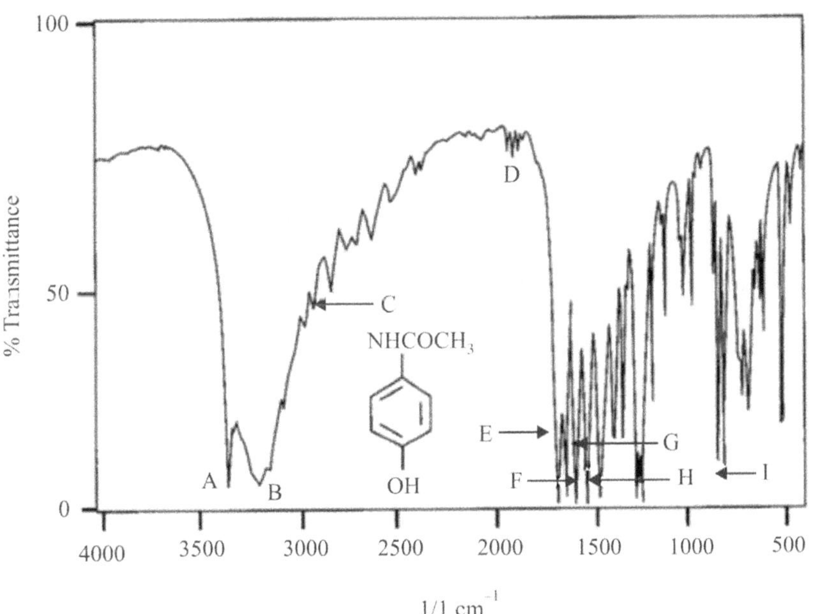

Observation Table

Peak No.	Wavenumber	Assignment	Comments
A	3360 cm^{-1}	N-H amide stretch	This band can be seen quite clearly although it is on top of the broad OH stretch
B	3000-3500 cm^{-1}	Phenolic OH stretch	Very broad due to strong hydrogen bonding and thus hide other bands in this region
C	3000 cm^{-1}	C-H stretching	Not clear due to underlying OH absorption
D	1840-1940 cm^{-1}	Aromatic overtone region	Quite clear fingerprint but does not reflect
E	1650 cm^{-1}	C=O amide stretch	C=O stretching in amides occurs at a low wavenumber compared to other unconjugated C=O groups
F	1608 cm^{-1}	Aromatic C=C stretch	This band is strong since the aromatic ring has polar substituents which increase the dipole moment of the C=C bonds in the ring
G	1568 cm^{-1}	N-H amide bending	Strong absorption in this case but not always so
H	1510 cm^{-1}	Aromatic C=C stretch	Evidence of a doublet due to interaction with ring substituents
I	810 cm^{-1}	=C-H bending	Possibly aromatic C-H bending but the fingerprint region is too complex to be completely confident of the assignment

Experiment 20.2

To Interpret IR Spectra of Aspirin

Theory

Aspirin, also known as **acetylsalicylic acid,** is a salicylate and a nonsteroidal anti-inflammatory drug (NSAID). Aspirin causes several different effects in the body, mainly the reduction of inflammation, analgesia (relief of pain), the prevention of clotting, and the reduction of fever. Much of this is believed to be due to decreased production of prostaglandins and TXA2. Aspirin's ability to suppress the production of prostaglandins and thromboxanes is due to its irreversible inactivation of the cyclooxygenase (COX) enzyme. Cyclooxygenase is required for prostaglandin and thromboxane synthesis. Aspirin is used to reduce fever and relieve mild to moderate pain from conditions such as muscle aches, toothaches, common cold, and headaches. It may also be used to reduce pain and swelling in conditions such as arthritis.

Spectra of Aspirin

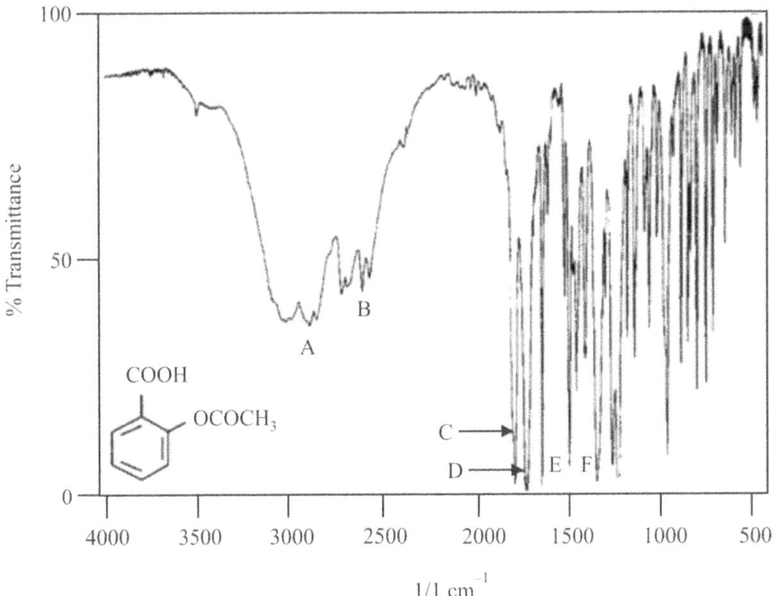

Observation Table

Peak No.	Wavenumber	Inference	Comments
A	2400-3300 cm^{-1}	Carboxylic OH stretch	Very broad peak and complex due to strong hydrogen bonding. The broad band obscures other bands in this region
B	3000 cm^{-1}	C-H stretching	Not clear due to underlying OH absorption
C	1757 cm^{-1}	C=O ester stretch	Due the acetyl group which is an un-conjugated aliphatic ester
D	1690 cm^{-1}	C=O ester stretch	C=O of the acid is conjugated to the aromatic ring
E	1608 cm^{-1}	Aromatic C=C stretch	These bands are intense since the ring substituted with polar groups
F	1460 cm^{-1}	Aromatic C=C stretch	

Experiment 20.3

To Interpret IR Spectra of Dexamethasone

Theory

Dexamethasone is a potent synthetic member of the glucocorticoid class of steroid drugs   that   has anti-inflammatory and immunosuppressant properties. It is 25 times more potent than cortisol in its glucocorticoid effect, while having minimal mineralocorticoid effect.

Spectra of Dexamethasone

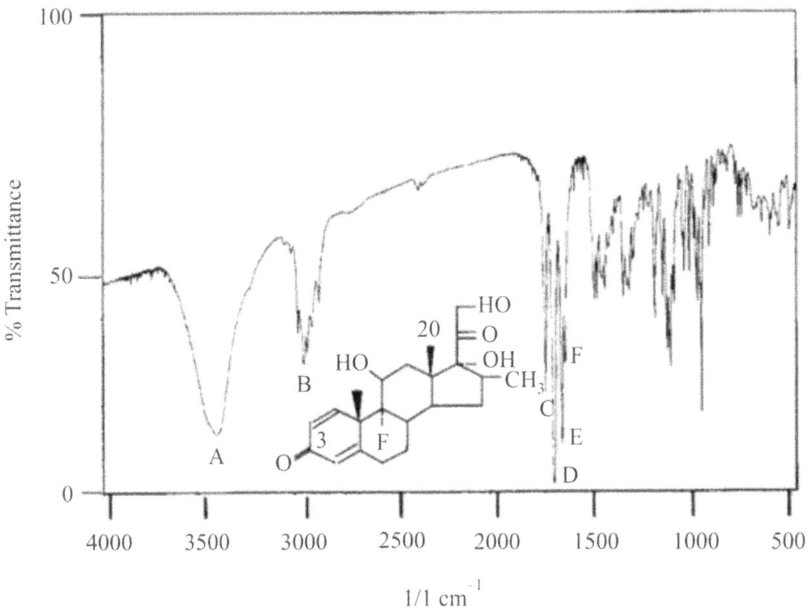

Observation Table

Peak No.	Wavenumber	Inference	Comments
A	3140-3600 cm^{-1}	Alcoholic OH stretch	Peak is broad due to hydrogen bonding
B	2750-3122 cm^{-1}	C-H stretching	The region is complex due to the large hydrocarbon structure of steroid
C	1705 cm^{-1}	C=O unconjugated ketone stretch	C=O stretch of ketone at 20-position appears at a lower wavenumber than ester
D	1655 cm^{-1}	C=O conjugated ketone stretch	Stretch due to ketone at 3-position
E	1615 cm^{-1}	C=C conjugation	Strengthened by being conjugated to C=O group. Trisubstituted C=C absorbs at higher wavenumber than disubstituted
F	1600 cm^{-1}	C=C conjugation	Strengthened by being conjugated to C=O group. Disubstituted C=C absorbs at lower wavenumber than trisubstituted

Experiment 20.4

To Interpret IR Spectra of Stigmasterol

Theory

Stigmasterol is an unsaturated plant sterol occurring in the plant fats or oils of soybean, calabar bean, and rape seed, and in a number of medicinal herbs, including the Chinese herbs *Ophiopogon japonicus* (Mai men dong) and American Ginseng. Stigmasterol is also found in various vegetables, legumes, nuts, seeds and unpasteurized milk. Soybean stigmasterol is used as a precursor in the manufacture of semisynthetic progesterone, a valuable human hormone that plays an important physiological role in the regulatory and tissue rebuilding mechanisms related to estrogen effects, as well as acting as an intermediate in the biosynthesis of androgens, estrogens, and corticoids. It is also used as the precursor of vitamin D_3.

Spectra of Stigmasterol

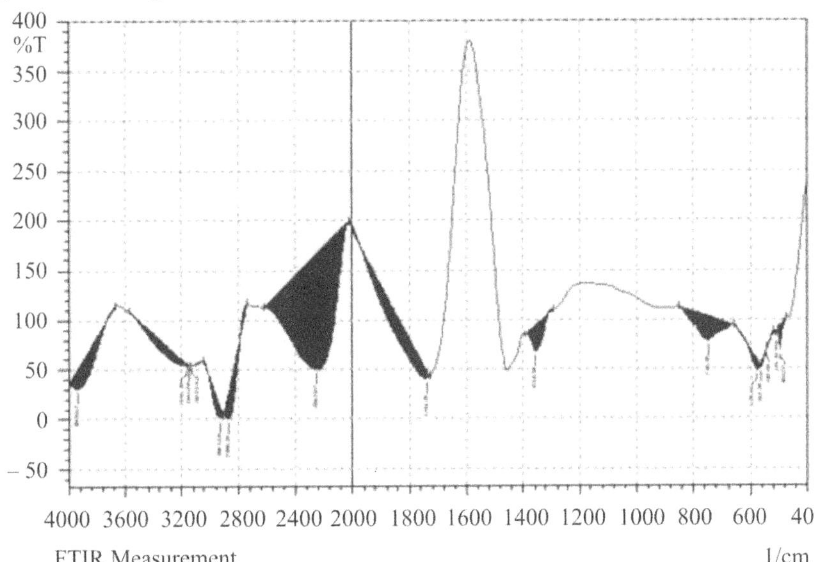

Observation table

Peak No.	Wavenumber	Inference	Comments
A	3185 cm^{-1}	OH stretch	Peak is broad due to hydrogen bonding
B	2891-3128 cm^{-1}	C-H aliphatic stretch	The region is complex due to the large hydrocarbon structure of steroid
C	1747 cm^{-1}	C=C stretch	Ring tension shifts the absorption to left
D	1445 cm^{-1}	CH$_3$ bend	Aliphatic bending
E	1354 cm^{-1}	CH$_2$ bend	Bending of substituted aliphatic group
F	748.38 cm^{-1}	CH bend (alkenes)	Due to the presence of long aliphatic chain

Experiment 20.5

To Interpret IR Spectra of Phenoxymethyl Penicillin Potassium

Theory

Phenoxymethylpenicillin, commonly known as penicillin V, is a penicillin antibiotic that is orally active. It is less active than benzyl-penicillin (penicillin G) against Gram-negative bacteria. Phenoxymethyl-penicillin is more acid-stable than benzylpenicillin, which allows it to be given orally. It exerts a bactericidal action against penicillin-sensitive microorganisms during the stage of active multiplication. It acts by inhibiting the biosynthesis of cell-wall peptidoglycan. Phenoxy-methylpenicillin is usually used only for the treatment of mild to moderate infections and not for severe or deep-seated infections since absorption can be unpredictable.

Spectra of Phenoxymethyl penicillin potassium

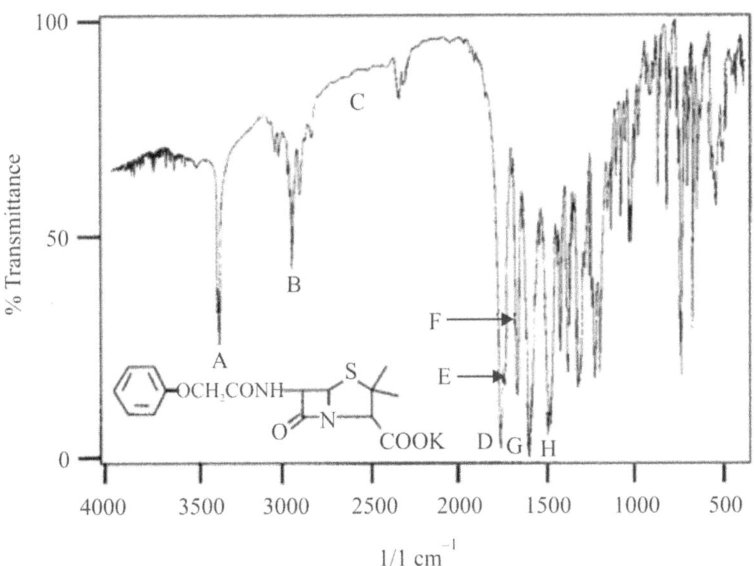

Observation table

Peak No.	Wavenumber	Inference	Comments
A	3360 cm^{-1}	N-H amide stretch	Two bands appear indicating restricted rotation about N-CO bond resulting in stereoisomers
B	2900-3100 cm^{-1}	C-H stretch	Aliphatic and aromatic C-H stretching. OH stretch is absent due to the presence of potassium salt form of carboxylic acid
C	2400-3000 cm^{-1}	C-H stretch	
D	1765 cm^{-1}	C=O lactam ring stretch	High energy C=O stretch is typical for lactam ring
E	1744 cm^{-1}	C=O carboxylic acid stretch	Salt form leads to the higher energy stretch than acid
F	1690 cm^{-1}	C=O amide stretch	Aromatic ring stretch, broad band possibly obscuring amide N-H bend
G	1610 cm^{-1}	C=C stretch	
H	1505 and 1495 cm^{-1}	C=C stretch	Due to aromatic ring

CHAPTER 21

High Performance Liquid Chromatography

High-performance liquid chromatography (or High pressure liquid chromatography, HPLC) is a specific form of column chromatography generally used in biochemistry and analysis to separate, identify and quantify the active compounds. Chromatography is the most frequently used analytical technique in pharmaceutical analysis. An understanding of the parameters which govern chromatographic performance has given rise to improvements in chromatographic systems so that the ability to achieve high resolution separations is continually increasing. High performance liquid chromatography (HPLC) is the technique most commonly used for the quantitation of drugs in formulations. The technique is called high performance because of the improved performance in comparison to conventional column chromatography (Table 21.1). It is also called high pressure liquid chromatography sine high pressure is used.

Table 21.1 Comparison of classical column chromatography with HPLC

Parameter	Classical Column chromatography	HPLC
Stationary phase	Large 60–200 μ	Small 3-20 μ
Column size Length × internal diameter	Large 0.5-5 m × 0.5-5 cm i.d.	Small 5-50 cm × 1-10 mm i.d.
Column material	Glass	Mostly metal
Column packing pressure	Slurry packed at low pressure-often gravity	Slurry packed at high pressure > 5000 psi
Operating pressure	Low (20 psi)	High (500-3000 psi)
Flow rates	Low to very low	Medium-High
Sample load	Low to medium (g/mg)	Low or very low (μg)
Column efficiency *i.e.* resolving power	(Low) < 500-theoretical plates per meter	(High) often > 1,00,000-theoretical plates per meter
Cost	Low-few hundreds	High-few lacs

Table 21.1 *Contd...*

Parameter	Classical Column chromatography	HPLC
Detector flow cell volume	Large-300-1000 μL	Low 2-10 μL
Types of stationary phases available	Limited range	Wide range
Scale of operation	Preparative scale	Analytical and preparative scale

Principle

A liquid mobile phase is pumped under pressure through a stainless steel column containing particles of stationary phase with a diameter of 3-10 μm. The analyte is loaded onto the head of the column *via* a loop valve and separation of a mixture occurs according to the relative lengths of time spent by its components in the stationary phase. It should be noted that all components in a mixture spend more or less the same time in the mobile phase in order to exit the column. Monitoring of the column effluent can be carried out with a variety of detectors.

Types of HPLC techniques

- ***Based on modes of chromatography:*** There are two modes viz. Normal phase and Reverse phase.

- ***Normal phase:*** In normal phase mode, the stationary phase is polar (e.g., silica gel) in nature and the mobile phase is non-polar. In this technique non-polar compounds travel faster and are eluted first. This is because of less affinity with the polar stationary phase. Polar compounds are retained in the column for longer time because of more affinity towards the stationary phase. This is not advantageous in pharmaceutical applications since most drug molecules are polar in nature.

- ***Reverse phase:*** In reverse phase technique, stationary phase is non-polar and the mobile phase is polar in nature. In this mode, polar compounds are eluted first due to their less affinity towards stationary phase followed by non-polar components. Since most drugs are polar they are eluted faster, which is advantageous.

- ***Size exclusion chromatography:*** Size exclusion chromatography (SEC), also called as gel permeation chromatography or gel filtration chromatography mainly separates particles on the basis of size. It is also useful for determining the tertiary structure and quaternary structure of proteins and amino acids. This technique is widely used for the molecular weight determination of polysaccharides.

- *Ion exchange chromatography:* In Ion-exchange chromatography, retention is based on the attraction between solute ions and charged sites bound to the stationary phase. Ions of the same charge are excluded. This form of chromatography is widely used in purifying water, Ligand-exchange chromatography, Ion-exchange chromateography of proteins, High-pH anion-exchange chromatography of carbohydrates and oligosaccharides, etc. [3, 4]

- *Bio-affinity chromatography:* Separation based on specific reversible interaction of proteins with ligands. Ligands are covalently attached to solid support on a bio-affinity matrix, retains proteins with interaction to the column-bound ligands. Proteins bound to a bioaffinity column can be eluted in two ways:

- *Biospecific elution:* inclusion of free ligand in elution buffer which competes with column bound ligand.

- *Aspecific elution:* change in pH, salt, etc. which weakens interaction protein with column-bound substrate.

- Because of specificity of the interaction, bioaffinity chromatography can result in very high purification in a single step (10 - 1000-fold).

Based on elution technique

- *Isocratic separation:* In this technique, the same mobile phase combination is used throughout the process of separation.

- *Gradient elution:* In this technique, a mobile phase combination of lower polarity or elution strength is used followed by gradually increasing the polarity or elution strength.

Based on the scale of operation

- *Analytical HPLC,* where only analysis of the samples are done. Recovering of the samples for reuse is normally not done.

- *Preparative HPLC,* where the individual fractions of pure compounds can be collected using fraction collector. The collected samples are reused.

Based on the type of analysis

- *Qualitative analysis:* It is used to identify the compound, detect the presence of impurities, to find number of components etc. this is done by using retention time values.

- *Quantitative analysis:* It is used to determine the quantity of the component present in a mixture. This is done by comparing the peak area of the standard and the sample.

Instrumentation: The essential features of a modern HPLC (Figure 21.1) comprises of following basic components:

- *A solvent delivery system including pump*
- *Mixing unit, gradient controller and solvent degassing*
- *Sample injection system*
- *Guard column*
- *Analytical column*
- *A detector or recording system*

Solvent delivery system

The mobile phase is pumped under pressure (1000-6000 psi) from one or more reservoirs and flows through the column at a constant rate. This is because the particle size of the stationary phase is few μm, the resistance to the flow of solvent is high. Thus, such high pressure is recommended. The choice of mobile phase is very important in HPLC and the eluting power of the mobile phase is determined by its overall polarity, the polarity of the stationary phase and the nature of sample components. The solvents used must be of high purity, preferable HPLC grade.

There are different types of pumps available: mechanical pumps and pneumatic pumps. Mechanical pumps operate with constant flow rate and use sapphire piston. This type of pump is mainly used in analytical scale. Pneumatic pump operates with constant pressure and use highly compressed gas.

Mixing unit, gradient controller and solvent degassing

- ***Mixing unit:*** Mixing unit is used to mix solvents in different proportions and pass through the column. There are two types of mixing units:
- ***Low pressure mixing chamber*** which uses helium for degassing solvents.
- ***High pressure mixing chamber*** which uses static mixer or magnetic stirrer operating under high pressure.
- ***Gradient controller:*** In an isocratic separation, mobile phase is prepared by using pure solvent *i.e.,* same polarity is used. In gradient elution, the polarity of the solvent is increased gradually. Hence a gradient controller is used when two or more solvent pumps are used.

- ***Solvent degasser:*** When solvents are pumped under high pressure, gas bubbles are formed which interferes in the separation process. Hence degassing of the solvent is done by using one of the following techniques:

- ***Vacuum filtration:*** removes the air bubbles.

- ***Helium purging:*** by passing helium through the solvent. This is very effective method but helium is costly.

- ***Ultrasonication:*** by using ultrasonicator, this converts ultra high frequency to mechanical vibrations.

- ***Injector:*** Several devices are available either for manual or auto injection of the sample. Different devices are,

- ***Septum injectors:*** It is used for injecting the sample through a rubber septum. This is not common because the septum has to withstand high pressure.

- ***Stop flow:*** In this injector, the flow of mobile phase is stopped for a while and the sample is injected through a valve device.

- ***Rheodyne injector:*** It is the most popular injector. This has a fixed loop like 20 µL or 50 µL or more. Injector has two modes *i.e.*, **load position** when the sample is loaded in the loop and **inject mode** when the sample is injected.

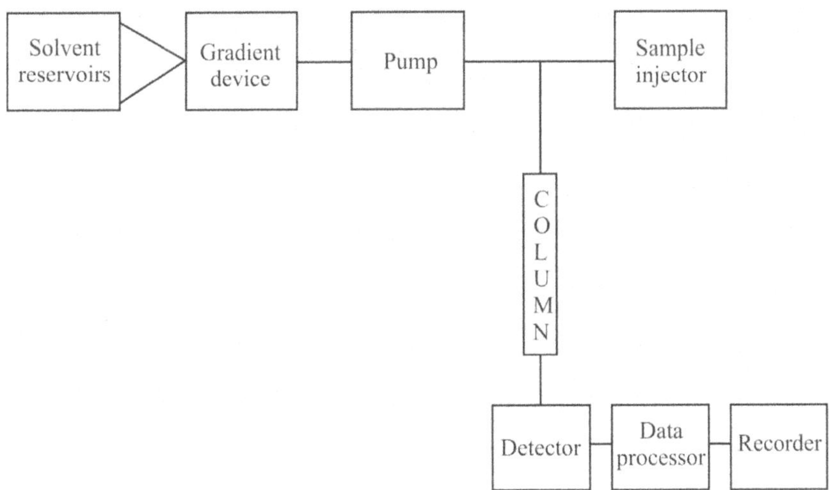

Fig. 21.1 Block diagram of HPLC.

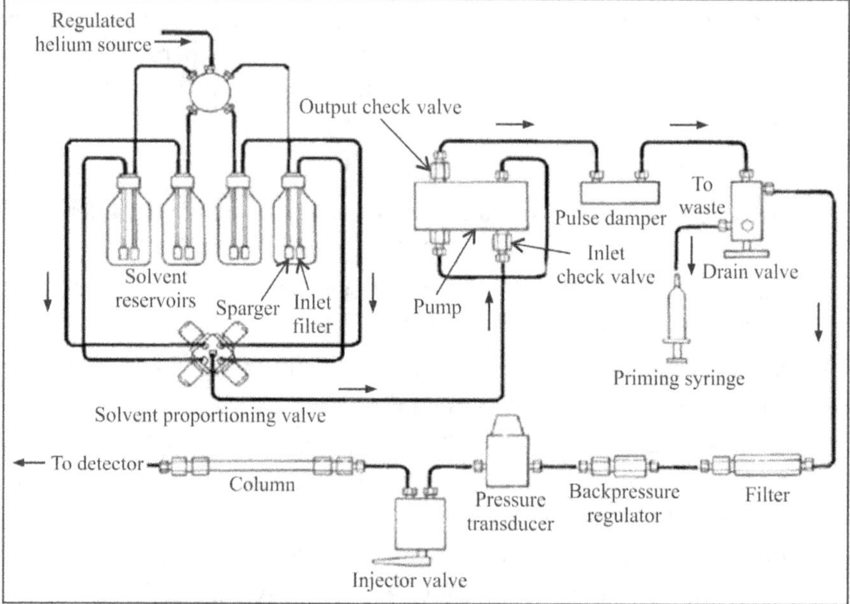

Guard column: It has very small quantity of adsorbent and improves the life of the analytical column. It also acts as a pre-filter to remove particulate matter. Guard column has the same material as that of the analytical column but it does not contribute to any separation.

- ***Analytical column:*** analytical column is the most important part of HPLC technique which decides the efficiency of separation. There are several stationary phases available depending upon the technique or mode of separation used (Table 21.2).

- ***Column material:*** The columns are made up of stainless steel, glass, polyethylene or PEEK (Poly ether ether ketone). Most widely used are stainless steel which can withstand high pressure.

Table 21.2 Some commonly used HPLC stationary phases

Stationary phase	Applications
ODS silica gel	The most commonly used phase, applicable to most problems in analysis of pharmaceutical formulations.
Octyl silane and butyl silane silica gels	Useful alternatives to ODS phases. The shorter hydrocarbon chains do not tend to lead to shorter retention times of analytes since the carbon loading on the surface of the silica gel may be higher for these phases and retention time is also dependant on how much the stationary phase is accessible to partitioning by the analyte.

Table 21.2 *Contd...*

Stationary phase	Applications
Phenyl silane silica gel	Useful for slightly more selective analytes of compounds containing large number of aromatic rings e.g., propranolol and naproxen.
Silica gel	Useful for chromatography of very lipophilic compounds such as in the separation of different classes of lipids and in the analysis of surfactants.
Aminopropyl silica gel	A moderately polar phase often used for the analysis of sugars and surfactants.
Cyanopropyl silica gel	A moderately polar phase applicable to the analysis of surfactants

- *Detectors:* **Detectors used depends upon the property of the compounds to be separated. Different detectors available are:**

- *UV-detector:* This detector is based upon the light absorption characteristics of the sample. Two types of this detector are available: **fixed wavelength detectors** which operate at 254 nm where most drugs absorb and **variable wavelength** detectors which can be operated from 900-1600 nm.

- *Refractive index detector:* This is a non specific or universal detector. This is not much used for analytical applications because of low sensitivity and specificity.

- *Fluorimetric detector:* This detector is based on the fluorescent radiation emitted by some class of compounds. The excitation wavelength and emission wavelength can be selected for each compound. This detector is more sensitive and specific.

- *Conductivity detector:* Based upon electrical conductivity the response is recorded. This detector is used when the sample has conducting ions like anions and cations.

- *Amperometric detector:* This detector is based on the reduction or oxidation of the compounds when a potential is applied. The diffusion current recorded is proportional to the concentration of the compound eluted. This is applicable when compounds have functional groups which can be either oxidized or reduced. This is a highly sensitive detector.

- *Photodiode array detector:* This detector is similar to UV detector which operates from 190-600 nm. Radiations of all wavelengths fall on the detector simultaneously. The resulting spectra if a three dimensional plot of Response *vs* Time *vs* Wavelength. The advantage is that the wavelength need not be selected.

- ***Recording system:*** Recorders are used to record the responses obtained from detectors after amplification. They record the baseline and all the peaks obtained, with respect to time. Retention time for all the peaks can be find out from such recordings but the area of individual peaks cannot be known. An improved version of recorders is integrators. They record the individual peaks with retention time, height and width of the peaks, peak area and percentage of area etc. integrators provide more information on peaks than recorders. Computers and printers are used now days for recording and processing the data obtained.

- ***Applications***

- ***Chemical Separations:*** It is based on the fact that certain compounds have different migration rates given a particular column and mobile phase, the extent or degree of separation is mostly determined by the choice of stationary phase and mobile phase.

- ***Purification:*** Purification is defined as the process of separating or extracting the target compound from a mixture of compounds or contaminants. Each compound showed a characteristic peak under certain chromatographic conditions. The migration of the compounds and contaminants through the column need to differ enough so that the pure desired compound can be collected or extracted without incurring any other undesired compound.

- ***Identification:*** Generally assay of compounds are carried using HPLC. The parameters of this assay should be such that a clean peak of the known sample is observed from the chromatograph. The identifying peak should have a reasonable retention time and should be well separated from extraneous peaks at the detection levels which the assay will be performed. The combination of HPLC with monitoring by UV/visible detection provides an accurate, precise and robust method for quantitative analysis of pharmaceutical products and is the industry standard method for this purpose.

- Monitoring of the stability of pure drug substances and in drugs in formulations with quantitation of any degradation products.

- Measurement of drugs and their metabolites in biological fluids.

- Determination of partition coefficient and pKa values of drugs and of drug protein binding.

- *Pharmaceutical applications*
  - Pharmaceutical quality control and identification of active ingredients of dosage forms Tablet dissolution study and shelf-life determinations of pharmaceutical dosages form.
- *Clinical applications*
  - Quantification of ions in human urine Analysis of antibiotics in blood plasma.
  - Estimation of bilirubin and bilivirdin in blood plasma in case of hepatic disorders.
  - Detection of endogenous neuropeptides in extracellular fluids of brain.
- *Environmental applications*
  - Detection of phenolic compounds in Drinking Water.
  - Identification of diphenhydramine in sedimented samples.
  - Bio-monitoring of pollutant.
- *Forensics*
  - Identification of anabolic steroids in serum, urine, sweat, and hair.
  - Forensic analysis of textile dyes.
  - Quantification of the drug in biological samples.
- *Strengths*

  Easily controlled and precise sample introduction ensures quantitative precision.

  HPLC is the chromatographic technique which has seen the most intensive development in recent years leading to improved, columns, detectors and software control.

  The variety of columns and detectors means that the selectivity of the method can be readily adjusted.

  Compared to gas chromatography there is risk of sample degradation because heating is not required in the chromatographic process.

Readily automated

Limitations: There is still a requirement for reliable and inexpensive detectors which can monitor compounds that lack a chromophore.

Drugs have to be extracted from their formulations prior to analysis.

Large amounts of organic solvent waste are generated, which is expensive to dispose of.

Spectra of some compounds eluted using HPLC:

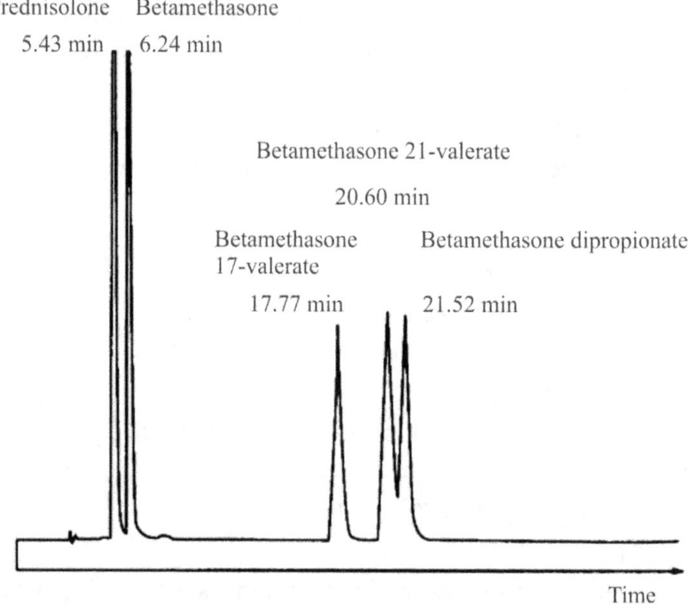

Fig. 21.2 Prednisolone and betamethasone and their esters eluted from ODS column with methanol:water (75:25) as mobile phase and UV detection at 240 nm.

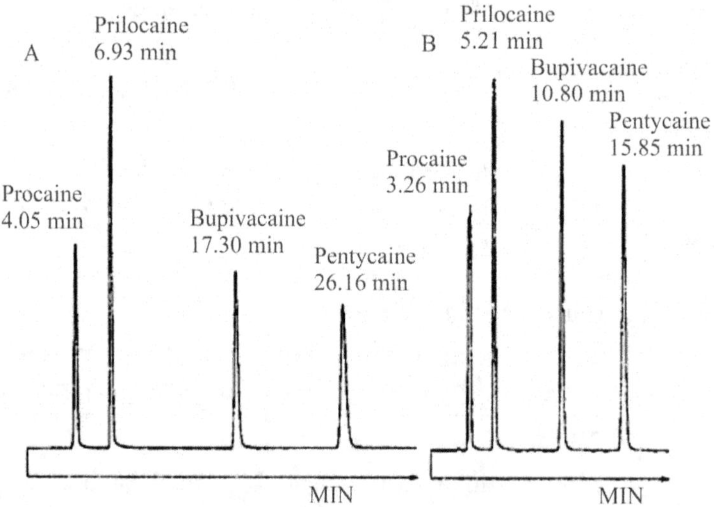

Fig. 21.3 Some local anesthetics eluted from an ODS column with (A) acetonitrile/TRIS. HCl buffer pH 8.4 (60:40) and (B) acetonitrile/TRIS. HCl buffer pH 7.4 (60:40).

Experiment 21.1

Assay of Paracetamol and Aspirin in Tablets

Aim

Assay of paracetamol and aspirin in tablets

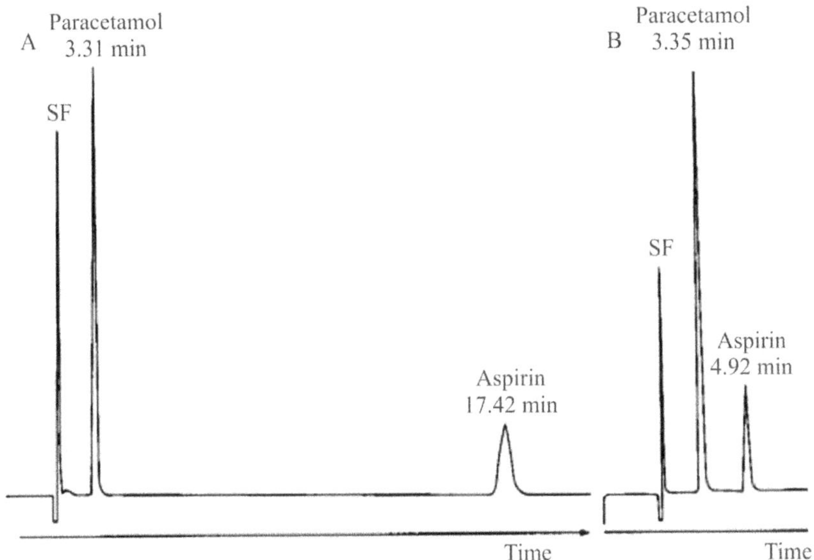

Fig. 21.4 (A) A tablet extract containing paracetamol and aspirin run at a pH of 3.7 in 0.05 M acetic acid/acetonitrile (85:15) (150 mm × 4.6 mm ODS column, flow rate 1 mL/min), (B) shows the tablets extract run at pH 4.4 in 0.05 M sodium acetate buffer/acetonitrile (85:15). ODS column 150 mm × 4.6 mm, flow rate 1 mL/min. UV detection at 243 nm.

Data obtained

- Weight of 20 tablets = 11.2698 g
- Weight of tablet powder taken = 283.8 mg

- Weight of paracetamol standard = 125.5 mg
- Weight of aspirin standard = 127.3 mg

Mean area of chromatographic peaks for a duplicate analysis of the tablet extract:

- Aspirin = 15366
- Paracetamol = 44535

The equations for the calibration lines obtained were as follows:

- Aspirin: $y = 12136\,x + 139$
- Paracetamol: $y = 35374\,x - 35$